VEGETARIAN DIET

COMPREHENSIVE GUIDE AND COOKBOOK FOR FOLLOWING THE VEGETARIAN DIET WITH RECIPES SPECIFIC TO THE MALE BODY AND HELPING TO IMPROVE HEALTH AND LOSE WEIGHT

By

Jim MOON

© Copyright 2021 - All rights reserved.

The content contained within this book may not be reproduced, duplicated or transmitted without direct written permission from the author or the publisher.

Under no circumstances will any blame or legal responsibility be held against the publisher, or author, for any damages, reparation, or monetary loss due to the information contained within this book. Either directly or indirectly.

Legal Notice:

This book is copyright protected. This book is only for personal use. You cannot amend, distribute, sell, use, quote or paraphrase any part, or the content within this book, without the consent of the author or publisher.

Disclaimer Notice:

Please note the information contained within this document is for educational and entertainment purposes only. All effort has been executed to present accurate, up to date, and reliable, complete information. No warranties of any kind are declared or implied. Readers acknowledge that the author is not engaging in the rendering of legal, financial, medical or professional advice. The content within this book has been derived from various sources. Please consult a licensed professional before attempting any techniques outlined in this book.

By reading this document, the reader agrees that under no circumstances is the author responsible for any losses, direct or indirect, which are incurred as a result of the use of information contained within this document, including, but not limited to, — errors, omissions, or inaccuracies.

TABLE OF CONTENS
VEGETARIAN DIET GUIDE 5
HEALTH BENEFITS OF VEGETARIAN DIET 5
WHAT TO EAT: MACRO- AND MICRO-NUTRIENTS... 5
HOW TO CHOOSE THE RIGHT FOOD FOR VEGETARIAN 7
BREAKFAST RECIPES 9
   1)   SPINACH SALAD 10
   2)   ZUCCHINI BUTTER 10
   3)   OREGANO PEPPERS BAKE 10
   4)   ASPARAGUS AND AVOCADO BOWLS 10
   5)   BERRY AND DATES OATMEAL 11
   6)   TOMATO OATMEAL 11
   7)   BREAKFAST BLUEBERRY MUFFINS 11
   8)   OATMEAL WITH PEARS 11
   9)   YOGURT WITH CUCUMBER 12
   10)   BREAKFAST CASSEROLE 12
   11)   COURGETTE RISOTTO 12
   12)   COUNTRY BREAKFAST CEREAL 13
   13)   OATMEAL FRUIT SHAKE 13
   14)   AMARANTH BANANA BREAKFAST PORRIDGE 13
   15)   GREEN GINGER SMOOTHIE 13
   16)   ORANGE DREAM CREAMSICLE 14
   17)   STRAWBERRY LIMEADE 14
   18)   TOMATO AND ZUCCHINI FRITTERS 14
   19)   PEPPERS CASSEROLE 15
   20)   LEEKS SPREAD 15
LUNCH RECIPES 16
   21)   AVOCADO, ENDIVE AND ASPARAGUS MIX 17
   22)   BELL PEPPERS AND SPINACH PAN 17
   23)   MUSHROOMS AND ASPARAGUS MIX 17
   24)   KALE AND RAISINS 17
   25)   COLLARD GREENS AND GARLIC MIX 18
   26)   CAULIFLOWER RICE AND CHIA MIX 18
   27)   FRUITY CAULIFLOWER RICE BOWLS 18
   28)   SPICY ASIAN BROCCOLI 18
   29)   TOMATO CUCUMBER CHEESE SALAD 19
   30)   HEALTHY BRUSSELS SPROUT SALAD 19
   31)   HEALTHY BRAISED GARLIC KALE 19
   32)   CAULIFLOWER LATKE 19
   33)   ROASTED BRUSSELS SPROUTS 20
   34)   BRUSSELS SPROUTS & CRANBERRIES SALAD 20
   35)   POTATO LATKE 20
   36)   BROCCOLI RABE 21
   37)   WHIPPED POTATOES 21
   38)   QUINOA AVOCADO SALAD 21
   39)   ROASTED SWEET POTATOES 22
   40)   CAULIFLOWER SALAD 22
SNACK RECIPES 23
   41)   CANDIED ALMONDS 24
   42)   STUFFED MUSHROOMS 24
   43)   KETTLE CORN 24
   44)   BLOOMING ONION 25
   45)   BRUSCHETTA 25
   46)   SPICY JALAPEÑO POPPERS 25
   47)   MEXICAN ROLL-UPS 26
   48)   BAKED ZUCCHINI 26
   49)   PUMPKIN SEEDS 26
   50)   SPINACH BARS 27
   51)   QUINOA BROCCOLI TOTS 27
   52)   SPICY ROASTED CHICKPEAS 27

53)	NACHO KALE CHIPS	28
54)	RED SALSA	28
55)	TOMATO HUMMUS	28
56)	MARINATED MUSHROOMS	29
57)	HUMMUS QUESADILLAS	29
58)	NACHO CHEESE SAUCE	29
59)	AVOCADO TOMATO BRUSCHETTA	30
60)	CINNAMON BANANAS	30

DINNER RECIPES 31

61)	GINGER LIME TEMPEH	32
62)	TOFU MOZZARELLA	32
63)	SEITAN MEATZA WITH KALE	33
64)	TACO TEMPEH CASSEROLE	33
65)	BROCCOLI TEMPEH ALFREDO	34
66)	AVOCADO SEITAN	34
67)	SEITAN MUSHROOM BURGERS	35
68)	TACO TEMPEH STUFFED PEPPERS	35
69)	TANGY TOFU MEATLOAF	36
70)	VEGAN BACON WRAPPED TOFU WITH BUTTERED SPINACH	36
71)	CAULIFLOWER MIX	36
72)	BAKED BROCCOLI AND PINE NUTS	37
73)	CHILI ASPARAGUS	37
74)	TOMATO QUINOA	37
75)	CORIANDER BLACK BEANS	37
76)	GREEN BEANS AND MANGO MIX	38
77)	QUINOA WITH OLIVES	38
78)	GARLIC ASPARAGUS AND TOMATOES	38
79)	HOT CUCUMBER MIX	39
80)	TOMATO SALAD	39

DESSERT RECIPES 40

81)	CHOCOLATE WATERMELON CUPS	41
82)	VANILLA RASPBERRIES MIX	41
83)	COCONUT SALAD	41
84)	MINT COOKIES	41
85)	MINT AVOCADO BARS	42
86)	COCONUT CHOCOLATE CAKE	42
87)	MINT CHOCOLATE CREAM	42
88)	CRANBERRIES CAKE	43
89)	SWEET ZUCCHINI BUNS	43
90)	LIME CUSTARD	43
91)	CANDIED PECANS	44
92)	RICE AND CANTALOUPE RAMEKINS	44
93)	STRAWBERRIES CREAM	44
94)	ALMOND AND CHIA PUDDING	45
95)	DATES AND COCOA BOWLS	45
96)	NUTS AND SEEDS PUDDING	45
97)	CASHEW FUDGE	46
98)	LIME BERRIES STEW	46
99)	APRICOTS CAKE	46
100)	BERRY CAKE	47

VEGETARIAN DIET GUIDE
HEALTH BENEFITS OF VEGETARIAN DIET

I've already mentioned some of the health benefits but let me back it up with some science. Of course, as mentioned earlier, if you eat only processed foods packed with sugar and saturated and trans-fat, eat little to no vegetables and fruits, and don't meet your macronutrient targets, you won't reap the benefits.

Boosts Heart Health
Following a plant-based diet makes you up to one-third less likely to end up in the hospital or die due to heart disease (Crowe et al., 2013). It all comes down to eating foods that will keep your blood sugar levels stable. High-fiber whole grains, nuts, legumes, and low-glycemic foods, in general, will reduce your overall risk of heart disease and lower your cholesterol (Harvard Medical School, 2020).

Reduces Cancer Risk
Vegetarians may have the upper hand when it comes to fighting off cancer (Tantamango-Bartley et al., 2013). This study found that plant-based diets don't only reduce your overall risk for cancer more than other diets; it is also more effective against female-specific cancers. Also, when it comes to Lacto- ovo vegetarians, they have a smaller chance of getting cancers of the gastrointestinal tract.
The consensus is that a diet filled with fresh fruits and veggies is key to combating cancer, and, of course, being a vegetarian makes it easier for you to get the recommended five servings a day.
Although the benefit isn't that significant, it is worth mentioning since every bit helps in the fight against the "big C."

Prevents Type 2 Diabetes
Following a healthy plant-based diet may prevent type 2 diabetes (Chiu et al., 2018). In fact, you have half the risk of developing this disease (Tonstad et al., 2013), and the good news doesn't stop there. If you already suffer from this disease, a vegetarian diet will help treat the associated symptoms and may even reverse the disease entirely (Jenkins et al., 2003).
Eating foods that keep your blood sugar levels steady is the secret behind preventing type 2 diabetes—something you'll be doing a lot of when you follow a vegetarian diet.

Lowers Blood Pressure
Plant foods are lower in fat and contain less sodium and cholesterol, which means they will help lower your blood pressure. Furthermore, fruits and veggies contain high potassium concentrations, which also help to lower blood pressure. Studies show that following a plant-based diet, primarily vegan, leads to lower blood pressure than those who consume animal products (Appleby et al., 2002).

Helps with Asthma
Animal foods trigger an allergy or inflammatory response in the body, so removing these foods from your diet will have a positive impact overall. One study (albeit an older one) found 22 out of 24 participants were less dependent on their asthma medication after adopting the vegetarian lifestyle (Lindahl et al., 1985).

Improves Your Mood
A lot of factors come into play when it comes to your mood—what you eat, how active you are, as well as your sleeping pattern. Since animal products are chemical-laden, cutting them from your diet will have a mood-boosting effect.

Increases Energy Levels Elevated energy levels are one of the most celebrated changes I noticed after switching to a vegetarian diet. There aren't enough hours in the day, but when you follow a plant-based diet, you have enough energy to do everything, and then some. Fruits and vegetables are high in vitamins and antioxidants, and this will give you a significant energy boost. The fact that your digestion will also run better due to the increased fiber will add to your newly-found get-up-and-go attitude!

Supports Better Sleep
Meat is heavy and can slow down digestion. When your body doesn't need to digest such dense proteins, you'll enjoy a better night's sleep. The speedier breakdown of plant protein also means your body will get all the minerals it needs for some much-needed shuteye. Add to that the fact that most vegetarians generally lead a healthier lifestyle—drink less, don't smoke, exercise regularly, etc., and counting sheep will be a thing of the past.

Improve Bone Health Osteoporosis is a leading cause of bone weakness, and this is caused by the removal of calcium from the bone and eventually leading to a hole in the bone. This condition is greatly reduced in people with a vegetarian diet. Eating animal products can lead to osteoporosis by forcing calcium out of the bone and eventually leading to less bone mineral. Those are some pretty amazing health benefits, right? And they're not the only ones—more and more studies are coming out documenting the positive bodily changes you'll experience if you cut out meat. Even a little goes a long way if you don't want to go full-blown vegetarian, try to steer your diet in a direction where the focus is more on fruits and veggies and less on meat. The Mediterranean diet comes to mind here!

WHAT TO EAT: MACRO- AND MICRO-NUTRIENTS

Since the standard American diet is built around animal protein, it's hard for most people to understand how vegetarians who reduce the ingredients they consider essential to a healthy diet will get the nutrients their bodies need. In fact, saturated fat and trans-fat in animal protein, antibiotics, chemicals, cholesterol, etc. are all harmful to the human body. If you learn about this, you will have to change your thinking about eating again In order to scientifically adjust your eating habits, I hope you have an understanding of protein, carbohydrates and fats, and understand how each nutrient is essential to the function of the body.

The best macronutrient breakdown for a vegetarian diet is as follows:
25% protein
45% carbohydrates
30% fat

If you're not sure what this means, you will need to work out how many calories your body needs per day to function at an optimal level. This depends on your body shape, age, activity level, etc. There are various calorie counters online that will help you calculate your daily caloric needs. Once you have this number, you just divide it in the above percentages, and "Bob's your uncle," as they say!

You will find people who will tell you that the vegetarian diet is too high in carbs. Well, not all carbs are the same Let me break down the various macronutrients and how much you need to eat to stay healthy. Afterward, we will look closer at the micronutrients.

Protein

Many vegetarians, both new and old, always have to deal with the problem of getting enough protein in their diet. The most important part of this is the confusion of how to deal with the choice of protein.

We both understand that protein is an essential part of a person's balanced diet. And most of our protein as humans comes from animals. But where will you get your protein from if you can't rely on a thick slice of steak? The truth is there are good numbers of protein sources from plants. As vegetarians, we have access to a wider variety of proteins, such as:

Tofu is the most familiar source of non-meat protein for a lot of vegetarians but believe me; there are many others I have tried and which you can too. Cooked Lentils; Cooked Beans; Whole Grain Pasta; Nuts; Eggplant; Tofu; Ground Flaxseed; Mushroom; Cauliflower; and Cooked Quinoa are some of the best sources of plant protein that you can add to maintain a balanced meal

It should now be clear that the belief that plant-based protein won't be enough to sustain your body's protein needs is unfounded. Ultimately, the building blocks of both types of protein (amino acids) are the same—on a cellular level, your body won't be able to tell the difference. Furthermore, when your body breaks down the amino acids in the food, it will build complete proteins. This also smashes the myth that you'll need to eat various proteins in one sitting to 'mimic' animal protein.

Carbohydrates

As I mentioned before, not all carbohydrates are created equal. Our body needs carbohydrates to function properly, but you must choose the right type of carbohydrates to get the best results. When choosing carbohydrates, the more natural the ingredients, the better for the body, because the simplicity of processing and packaging contains almost no fiber. However, foods rich in plant fiber, vitamins, minerals and phytonutrients can help your body resist oxidation and inflammation. Fiber content can slow down the digestion of carbohydrates and control the rise of blood sugar in the body. Eating high- fiber carbohydrates regularly helps you prevent type 2 diabetes, fight cancer, and keep your body in good condition.

As you read above, 45 percent of your daily calories should go to carbohydrates. If you follow a 2,000-calorie diet, you'll be eating 225 grams of carbs a day. However, you may end up eating more on a vegetarian diet, then you need to keep an eye on your carb intake to prevent weight gain.

Fat

I know you've been told that fat makes fat and leads to high cholesterol actually, people have misunderstood the role of fat for a long time. What's more, fat plays a vital role in your health. Fat is essential for the absorption of fat-soluble vitamins, cell growth, hormone production, and digestion. Research showed that eating good fats (polyunsaturated and monounsaturated) can help lose weight, reduce inflammation, fight depression and anxiety, and improve your overall health (Manikam, 2008).

Now that you know the importance of fat, I will tell you how to meet your daily fat needs from a vegetarian diet. First of all, it needs to be clear where we get good fats? Some foods include avocado (20 grams per 100 grams), soybeans (3.3 grams per cup), olives (3.2 grams per 28 grams) and pumpkin seeds (14 grams per tablespoon), both are good sources of fat. Another important thing is how to control the intake of fat in daily cooking.

☐ Sauté food using water or vegetable broth. Make sure to check the liquid level frequently you don't want your food to burn. Just keep adding water or broth until your food is cooked. Fruit or vegetable purée and applesauce are great oil substitutes when you're baking. It will keep your cakes and other baked goods
moist.

☐ If you're grilling something in the oven, I highly recommend getting a silicone mat to line your pan with. You can also use parchment paper to create the perfect non-stick environment for your oil-free grilling.

☐ Invest in some non-stick cookware to help make cooking without oil less problematic. Okay, that covers your daily macronutrients. I think it's time we look at the vitamins and minerals (micronutrients) your body needs.

☐ Vitamins and Minerals

As I mentioned before and will highlight throughout this cookbook, you need to focus on eating a wide variety of whole grains, fruits, vegetables, and fats with a particular focus on meeting your protein target if you want to get in all the nutrients your body needs. However, there are some nutrients you'll have to pay extra attention, or even consider supplementing.

Vitamin B-12

I want to take a moment to focus on vitamin B-12—a vital nutrient, which isn't found in many plant foods. If you decide to cut out all animal food sources, then you will have to consume more vitamin B-12-rich foods or you will have to supplement this vitamin. Since B-12 plays an important role in producing red blood cells and preventing anemia, I recommend you add a supplement to your diet just to be safe.

Omega-3 Fatty Acids
Before we move on to healthy foods you can't go wrong eating daily, let's look at omega-3s. To boost the health benefits of the vegetarian diet, getting in a good dose of fatty acids like docosahexaenoic acid (DHA), Eicosapentaenoic acid (EPA), and alpha-linolenic acid (ALA) is a must! Omega-3s help combat inflammation in the body, and through doing that, decrease your risk of getting heart disease or other issues caused by inflamed cells. When I first heard omega-3, I immediately thought about seafood, but I was pleasantly surprised that you could find ALA in various vegetarian sources.

HOW TO CHOOSE THE RIGHT FOOD FOR VEGETARIAN

Although all fruits and vegetables are superfoods as they're packed with nutrients our bodies love, some do stand out above the rest. Since making the healthiest choices is what you should aim for when following a vegetarian diet, you can boost your success rate by eating specific fruits and veggies daily, as well as focusing on herbs, spices, and drinks that have proven benefits.
I'll share with you some of the foods I attempt to eat daily and others I pack on my plate at least once a week.
Daily
Berries
Berries aren't only delicious, they're some of the healthiest foods on the planet. The number of health benefits packed in these juicy snacks is impressive. Not only do they contain essential nutrients, but they're also chock full of antioxidants that help keep free radicals at bay. What's a free radical, you ask? Well, they're rogue and unstable molecules that do you good in small numbers but will cause oxidative stress when their numbers get too high (LiveScience, 2016). This increases your risk of getting various diseases. But thanks to blueberries, blackberries, and raspberries and their high antioxidant content (the highest out of all common fruits), you can protect your cells (Wolfe et al., 2008).
Leafy greens
Kale, spinach, chard, and arugula are s78ome of the leafy-green superstars out there. They're low in calories but packed with vitamins, phytonutrients, and fiber. They're good for you in more ways than you can imagine. If the bulk of the veggies you eat is green and leafy, you can be sure to feel like a new person—even your skin will glow.
Nuts and seeds
Nuts and seeds are tiny yet powerful sources of protein, fat, fiber, vitamins, and minerals. What I appreciate most about these snacks is that I feel full and stay satiated for longer after eating only a handful. It's the perfect "tie-me- over" food when your tummy starts to grumble.
Turmeric
You've probably read about the wonders of turmeric or, more specifically, the active compound curcumin. This spice has scientifically been proven to have remarkable health benefits ranging from preventing heart disease, degenerative brain diseases, and can even help combat cancer cells. Its anti- inflammatory and antioxidant properties make it an anti-aging super spice.
Beans
If you ask me, one of the most underrated foods out there. Not only are beans and legumes high in dietary fiber, protein, vitamins, and minerals, they also contain B vitamins that you need as much of as you can get. Evidence suggests that beans' high fiber content will improve cholesterol levels and help your gut stay in good shape. Again, it comes down to managing those blood sugar levels!
Onions and garlic
You may not consider onions and garlic as nutritional powerhouses, but I am happy to convince you otherwise. Onions are high in potassium, folate, vitamin B6, and vitamin C. Garlic, on the other hand, contains all the goodies onions do with thiamin, calcium, phosphorus, copper, and manganese added to the mix!
And don't forget that it makes almost all savory dishes taste better.
Green tea
This wonder beverage is one of the healthiest on the planet. It comes loaded with antioxidants, which, as we've established, is terrific news for your overall health. Some of the health benefits of green tea include improved brain function, lowered risk of heart disease, protection against cancer, and better weight management (Chacko et al., 2010).
Once a Week
Ginger
Ginger is used in traditional and alternative medicine the world over, primarily when it comes to digestive health and fighting off nasty germs. Gingerol is the active compound in ginger and is responsible for all the medicinal properties. What makes it so powerful is the anti-inflammatory and antioxidant effects it has. You read about free radicals and oxidative stress and accompanied diseases earlier on, and now you have another food source to help heal your body!
Lemon juice
One of the main reasons why I can't do without lemon juice may surprise you. No, it's not for its vitamin C content but for its ability to combat anemia! Since vegetarians are prone to iron deficiency, including lemon juice in our diet will help with iron absorption from plant sources (Ballot et al., 1987). Your gut can absorb iron from animal protein, but it has a hard time doing so from plant-based sources. So, to help your body out a little, add lemon to your diet, as well as vitamin C and citric acid.
Dark chocolate

Who wouldn't want to eat chocolate once a week? I am not talking about overly sweet, processed, milk chocolate but the real deal—dark chocolate. The more unrefined the chocolate, the higher its flavanol content, and that's what we want. Flavanols are good for your arteries, and that makes them great for your heart and overall body. It tells your arteries to relax, and that reduces your blood pressure (Schewe et al., 2008). If you can recall, I suffered from hypertension when I first started following a vegetarian diet. Finding out that dark chocolate could help was delightful news!

Dates

This is another antioxidant-packed food, but that's not the only reason why I enjoy it once a week or so—dates make an excellent natural sweetener. Since they're dried, their sugar content is higher than fresh fruit, making them the perfect substitute for white sugar. Not to mention that they'll add some extra nutrients and fiber to any recipe you're preparing!

I usually make a date paste (recipe included in this cookbook) and substitute one cup of sugar with one cup of date paste.

However, you have to keep in mind that dried fruit overall has a much higher calorie content than their fresh counterparts. Furthermore, most of these calories come from carbs. That's my way of suggesting you don't overdo it when you eat this super sweet food—the vitamin, mineral, protein, and fiber content should blind you to the fact that it is a high-calorie food.

By now, you can understand my obsession too. I can be more serious once it comes to my vegetarian diet. In the pages that follow, there are mouth-watering recipes that will make you wonder why you didn't go meat-free ages ago. I also include some meal plans—something I found invaluable when I first started following the vegetarian diet. It makes it possible for you to stick to your guns and learn as you go along.

Note: This book has given you all the information you need to do this diet correctly and do it right. It is essential to understand what you are getting into when you embark on this diet, and this book gave you valuable information that you can use to your advantage and avoid the problems that can come with this diet. You want to stay healthy and make sure that your body can do what it needs to do. As with anything, we emphasize that if something seems wrong or unnatural, you will need to see a doctor to make sure you are safe and that your body can handle this diet. Use the knowledge in this book to get amazing recipes and learn directions for excellent meals for yourself. Consult your doctor before to starting new diet.

BREAKFAST RECIPES

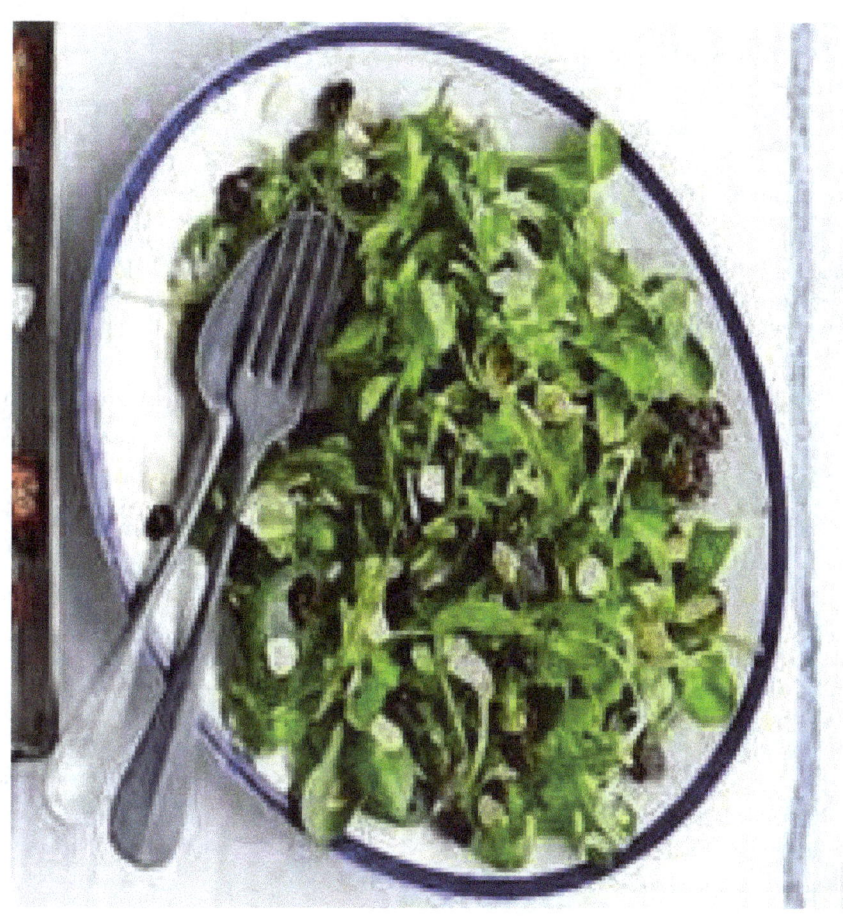

1) SPINACH SALAD

Preparation Time: 5 minutes **Cooking Time**: 0 minutes **Servings**: 2

Ingredients:
- 2 cups baby spinach
- 1 red bell pepper, roughly chopped
- 1 green bell pepper, roughly chopped
- ½ cup cherry tomatoes, halved
- 2 tablespoons olive oil

Ingredients:
- 1 teaspoon rosemary, dried
- 1 teaspoon basil, dried
- ½ teaspoon chili powder
- Salt and black pepper to the taste

Directions:
- In a bowl, combine the spinach with the peppers, tomatoes
- Add the other ingredients
- Toss and serve for breakfast.

2) ZUCCHINI BUTTER

Preparation Time: 10 minutes **Cooking Time**: 0 minutes **Servings**: 6

Ingredients:
- 3 tablespoons coconut oil, melted
- 1 pound zucchinis, grated
- 2 tablespoons coconut butter

Ingredients:
- A pinch of salt and black pepper
- 2 garlic cloves, minced
- 1 tablespoon chives, chopped

Directions:
- In a blender, combine the zucchinis with the coconut oil
- Add butter and the other Ingredients
- Pulse well. Divide into bowls and serve as a breakfast.

3) OREGANO PEPPERS BAKE

Preparation Time: 10 minutes **Cooking Time**: 40 minutes **Servings**: 4

Ingredients:
- ½ cup coconut milk
- 2 tablespoons flaxseed mixed with
- 3 tablespoons water
- Salt and black pepper to the taste
- 1 teaspoon oregano, dried
- 1 red bell pepper, cut into strips

Ingredients:
- 1 orange bell pepper, cut into strips
- 1 green bell pepper, cut into strips
- ½ cup chives, chopped
- 2 cups baby spinach
- Cooking spray

Directions:
- In a bowl, combine the peppers with the milk, flaxseed mix
- Then the other Ingredients except the cooking spray and stir.
- Grease a baking pan with the cooking spray
- Pour the peppers mix, spread and bake at 390 degrees F for 40 minutes.
- Divide the bake between plates and serve for breakfast.

4) ASPARAGUS AND AVOCADO BOWLS

Preparation Time: 5 minutes **Cooking Time**: 6 minutes **Servings**: 4

Ingredients:
- 1 tablespoon avocado oil
- 1 pound asparagus, trimmed and roughly sliced
- 2 avocados, peeled, pitted and sliced
- 2 tablespoons lemon juice

Ingredients:
- 1 tablespoon basil, chopped
- 2 teaspoons Dijon mustard
- 1 cup baby spinach
- Salt and black pepper to the taste

Directions:
- Heat up a pan with the oil over medium-high heat
- Add the asparagus, avocado, lemon juice and the other Ingredients
- Toss, cook for 6 minutes, divide into bowls and serve for breakfast

5) BERRY AND DATES OATMEAL

Preparation Time: 5 minutes   **Cooking Time:** 0 minutes   **Servings: 2**

Ingredients:
- ½ cup coconut flesh, unsweetened and shredded
- 1 cup coconut milk
- ¼ cup dates, chopped

Directions:
- In a bowl, combine the coconut flesh with the coconut milk

Ingredients:
- 1 teaspoon vanilla extract
- 1 tablespoon stevia
- 1 cup berries, mashed
- Add the dates and the other ingredients
- Whisk well, divide into 2 bowls and serve.

6) TOMATO OATMEAL

Preparation Time: 5 minutes   **Cooking Time:** 20 minutes   **Servings: 4**

Ingredients:
- 3 cups water
- 1 cup coconut milk
- 1 tablespoon avocado oil
- 1 cup coconut flesh, unsweetened and shredded

Directions:
- Meanwhile, heat up a pan with the oil over medium-high heat
- Add the tomatoes, chili powder and pepper flakes and sauté for 5 minutes
- Then the coconut and sauté for 5 minutes more.

Ingredients:
- ¼ cup cherry tomatoes, chopped
- A pinch of red pepper flakes
- 1 teaspoon chili powder
- Join also the remaining Ingredients, toss, bring to a simmer
- Cook over medium heat fro 10 minutes more
- Divide into bowls and serve for breakfast.

7) BREAKFAST BLUEBERRY MUFFINS

Preparation Time: 15 minutes   **Cooking Time:** 25 minutes   **Servings: 12**

Ingredients:
- Cooking spray
- 1 ½ cups rolled oats
- ¼ teaspoon baking soda
- 1 teaspoon baking powder
- ½ cup unsweetened applesauce
- ⅓ cup packed light brown sugar

Directions:
- Preheat your oven to 350 degrees F. Spray your muffin pan with oil.
- Add the oats in a food processor. Pulse until ground.
- Stir in the rest of the ingredients except blueberries. Pulse until smooth.

Ingredients:
- ¼ teaspoon salt
- 3 tablespoons vegetable oil
- 3 tablespoons water
- 1 tablespoon flax meal
- 1 teaspoon vanilla extract
- ¾ cup blueberries, sliced in half
- Pour the batter into the muffin pan. Top with the blueberries.
- Bake in the oven for 25 minutes. Store in a glass jar with lid.

8) OATMEAL WITH PEARS

Preparation Time: 15 minutes   **Cooking Time:** 15 minutes   **Servings: 1**

Ingredients:
- ¼ cup roll ed oats
- ¼ cup pear, sliced

Directions:
- Cook the oats according to the directions in the package.
- Stir in pear and ginger

Ingredients:
- 1/8 teaspoon ground ginger
- 1/8 teaspoon ground cinnamon
- Sprinkle with cinnamon
- Store in a glass jar with lid. Refrigerate overnight.

9) YOGURT WITH CUCUMBER

Preparation Time: 5 minutes **Cooking Time:** 0 minute **Servings: 1**

Ingredients:
- 1 cup soy yogurt
- ½ cucumber, diced
- ¼ teaspoon lemon zest

Directions:
- Put all the ingredients in a glass jar with lid

Ingredients:
- ¼ teaspoon freshly squeezed lemon juice
- Salt to taste
- Chopped mint leaves
- Refrigerate overnight or up to 2 days.

10) BREAKFAST CASSEROLE

Preparation Time: 20 minutes **Cooking Time:** 43 minutes **Servings: 6**

Ingredients:
- 10 oz. spinach
- 9 oz. artichoke hearts
- 2 cloves garlic, minced
- ¾ cup sun-dried tomatoes, chopped
- ½ teaspoon red pepper flakes

Directions:
- Squeeze the spinach to release the liquid. Add the spinach to a bowl.
- Stir in the artichoke hearts.
- In a pan over low heat, cook the garlic, tomatoes, red pepper
- Then lemon zest in oil for 3 minutes.
- Add the spinach and artichokes. Remove from heat.

Ingredients:
- 1 teaspoon lemon zest
- 1 tablespoon olive oil
- 2 cups almond milk
- 1 cup vegan cheese, crumbled
- 8 cups whole wheat bread, chopped
- Transfer to a baking pan.
- Stir in the spinach mixture and bread. Let sit for 30 minutes.
- Bake in the oven at 350 degrees F for 40 minutes
- Store in a food container and refrigerate.
- Reheat before serving.

11) COURGETTE RISOTTO

Preparation Time: 10 minutes **Cooking Time:** 5 minutes **Servings: 8**

Ingredients:
- 2 tablespoons olive oil
- 4 cloves garlic, finely chopped
- 1.5 pounds Arborio rice
- 6 tomatoes, chopped
- 2 teaspoons chopped rosemary
- 6 courgettes, finely diced

Directions:
- Place a large heavy bottomed pan over medium heat+ì
- Add oil. When the oil is heated, add onion and sauté until translucent.
- Stir in the tomatoes and cook until soft
- Next stir in the rice and rosemary. Mix well.

Ingredients:
- 1 ¼ cups peas, fresh or frozen
- 12 cups hot vegetable stock
- 1 cup chopped
- Salt to taste
- Freshly ground pepper
- Add half the stock and cook until dry
- Stir frequently. Add remaining stock and cook for 3-4 minutes.
- Then courgette and peas and cook until rice is tender
- Join also salt and pepper to taste.
- Stir in the basil. Let it sit for 5 minutes.

12) COUNTRY BREAKFAST CEREAL

Preparation Time: 5 minutes **Cooking Time:** 40 minutes **Servings: 6**

Ingredients:
- 1 cup brown rice, uncooked
- ½ cup raisins, seedless
- 1 tsp cinnamon, ground

Directions:
- ❖ Combine rice, butter, raisins, and cinnamon in a saucepan
- ❖ Add 2 ¼ cups water. Bring to boil.

Ingredients:
- ¼ Tbsp peanut butter
- 2 ¼ cups water Honey, to taste
- Nuts, toasted
- ❖ Simmer covered for 40 minutes until rice is tender
- ❖ Fluff with fork. Add honey and nuts to taste.

13) OATMEAL FRUIT SHAKE

Preparation Time: 10 minutes **Cooking Time:** 0 minutes **Servings: 2**

Ingredients:
- 1 cup oatmeal, already prepared, cooled
- 1 apple, cored, roughly chopped
- 1 banana, halved
- 1 cup baby spinach

Directions:
- ❖ Add all ingredients to a blender.

Ingredients:
- 2 cups coconut water
- 2 cups ice, cubed
- ½ tsp ground cinnamon
- 1 tsp pure vanilla extract
- ❖ Blend from low to high for several minutes until smooth.

14) AMARANTH BANANA BREAKFAST PORRIDGE

Preparation Time: 10 minutes **Cooking Time:** 25 minutes **Servings: 8**

Ingredients:
- 2 cup amaranth
- 2 cinnamon sticks
- 4 bananas, diced

Directions:
- ❖ Combine the amaranth, water, and cinnamon sticks, and banana in a pot

Ingredients:
- 2 Tbsp chopped pecans
- 4 cups water
- ❖ Cover and let simmer around 25 minutes.
- ❖ Remove from heat and discard the cinnamon. Places into bowls, and top with pecans.

15) GREEN GINGER SMOOTHIE

Preparation Time: 5 minutes **Cooking Time:** 5 minutes **Servings: 2**

Ingredients:
- 1 banana
- ½ apple sliced
- 1 orange sliced and peeled
- 1 lemon juice
- 2 big spinach

Directions:
- ❖ Take a blender. Peel off and slice all fruits
- ❖ Add banana, apple, orange, lime juice, ginger
- ❖ Then spinach and blend them well until they turn smooth
- ❖ Now add almond milk and pulse again for a few seconds

Ingredients:
- 1 tbsp. fresh ginger
- ½ cup almond milk
- For the dressing:
- Chia seeds, apple, raspberries
- ❖ Pour the smoothie into glasses and serve
- ❖ Add chia seeds, apple or raspberries for a smoothie bowl
- ❖ Store it up to 8-10 hours in the refrigerator.

16) ORANGE DREAM CREAMSICLE

Preparation Time: 5 minutes   **Cooking Time:** 5 minutes   **Servings: 2**

Ingredients:
- 1 orange, peeled
- ¼ cup vegan yogurt
- 2 tbsp. orange juice

Directions:
- In a blender, add orange, orange juice, vegan yogurt
- Then vanilla extract and ice cubes

Ingredients:
- ¼ tsp vanilla extract
- 4 ice cubes

- Blend all the ingredients well until smooth and well combined
- Pour it into smoothie glasses and serve.

17) STRAWBERRY LIMEADE

Preparation Time: 5 minutes   **Cooking Time:** 5 minutes   **Servings: 6**

Ingredients:
- 2 cup strawberries
- 1 cup sugar or as per taste
- 7 cups of water

Directions:
- Take a small bowl, add sugar and water and put in microwave until dissolved.
- Now take a blender and add strawberries and a cup of water and blend well.
- Combine the strawberries puree with the sugar dissolve water and mix

Ingredients:
- 2 cup lemon juice
- Sliced berries for garnish

- Pour lime juice and water if required
- Stir well and chill before serving
- You can add berries on the top as garnishing.

18) TOMATO AND ZUCCHINI FRITTERS

Preparation Time: 5 minutes   **Cooking Time:** 10 minutes   **Servings: 4**

Ingredients:
- 1 pound zucchinis, grated
- 2 tomatoes, cubed
- 2 garlic cloves, minced
- Salt and black pepper to the taste

Directions:
- In a bowl, mix the zucchinis with the tomatoes
- Add the other ingredients except the oil
- Stir well, shape medium fritters out of this mix and flatten them

Ingredients:
- 1 tablespoon coconut flour
- 1 tablespoon flaxseed mixed with 2 tablespoons water
- 1 tablespoon dill, chopped
- 2 tablespoons olive oil

- Heat up a pan with the oil over medium heat, add the fritters
- Cook them for 5 minutes on each side
- Divide between plates and serve for breakfast.

19) PEPPERS CASSEROLE

Preparation Time: 10 minutes **Cooking Time:** 25 minutes Servings: 4

Ingredients:
- 1 pound mixed bell peppers, cut into strips
- Salt and black pepper to the taste
- 4 scallions, chopped
- ½ teaspoon cumin, ground
- ½ teaspoon oregano, dried
- ½ teaspoon basil, dried

Ingredients:
- 2 garlic cloves, minced
- 1 tablespoon avocado oil
- 2 tomatoes, cubed
- 1.cup cashew cheese, grated
- 2.tablespoons parsley, chopped

Directions:
- Heat up a pan with the oil over medium heat
- Add the scallions and the garlic and sauté for 5 minutes.
- Theb the rest of the ingredients except the cheese
- Stir and cook for 5 minutes more.
- Sprinkle the cashew cheese on top
- Bake everything at 380 degrees F for 15 minutes.
- Divide the mix between plates and serve for breakfast.

20) LEEKS SPREAD

Preparation Time: 5 minutes **Cooking Time:** 10 minutes Servings: 4

Ingredients:
- 3 leeks, sliced
- 2 scallions, chopped
- 1 tablespoon avocado oil
- ¼ cup coconut cream

Ingredients:
- Salt and black pepper to the taste
- ¼ teaspoon garlic powder
- ½ teaspoon thyme, dried
- 1 tablespoon cilantro, chopped

Directions:
- Heat up a pan with the oil over medium heat
- Add the scallions and the leeks and sauté for 5 minutes.
- Then the rest of the ingredients
- Cook everything for 5 minutes more
- Blend using an immersion blender
- Divide into bowls and serve for breakfast.

LUNCH RECIPES

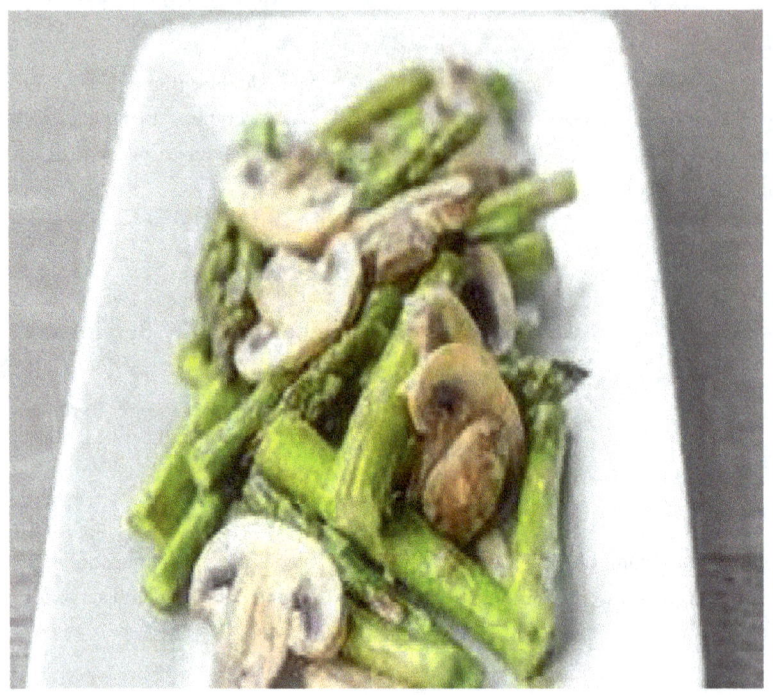

21) AVOCADO, ENDIVE AND ASPARAGUS MIX

Preparation Time: 10 minutes   **Cooking Time:** 10 minutes   **Servings: 4**

Ingredients:
- 3 avocados, peeled, pitted and sliced
- 2 endives, shredded
- 4 asparagus spears, trimmed and halved
- 2 tablespoons sesame seeds
- 2 tablespoons avocado oil

Directions:
- Heat up a pan with the oil over medium heat

Ingredients:
- Juice of 1 lime
- A pinch of sea salt and black pepper
- Black pepper to the taste
- 1 tablespoon chives, chopped

- Add the endives, asparagus, avocados and the other ingredients, toss
- Cook for 10 minutes, divide between plates and serve.

22) BELL PEPPERS AND SPINACH PAN

Preparation Time: 10 minutes   **Cooking Time:** 12 minutes   **Servings: 4**

Ingredients:
- 1 tablespoon olive oil
- 1 red bell pepper, cut into strips
- 1 green bell pepper, cut into strips
- 1 orange bell pepper, cut into strips
- 2 cups baby spinach

Directions:
- Heat up a pan with the oil over medium high heat
- Add the peppers and the garlic and sauté for 2 minutes.
- Then the spinach and the other Ingredients, toss

Ingredients:
- 3 garlic cloves, minced
- 2 teaspoons garlic powder
- A pinch of sea salt and black pepper
- 1 teaspoon fennel seeds, crushed
- 1 teaspoon chili powder

- Cook over medium heat for 10 minutes more
- Divide between plates and serve.

23) MUSHROOMS AND ASPARAGUS MIX

Preparation Time: 10 minutes   **Cooking Time:** 15 minutes   **Servings: 4**

Ingredients:
- 1 pound white mushrooms, sliced
- 1 asparagus bunch, trimmed and halved
- 1 teaspoon sweet paprika
- 1 teaspoon coriander, ground
- 1 teaspoon chili powder

Directions:
- Heat up a pan with the oil over medium high heat

Ingredients:
- ½ teaspoon thyme, dried
- 2 garlic cloves, minced
- ¼ cup coconut cream
- 1 tablespoon avocado oil

- Add the mushrooms, the asparagus and the other Ingredients, toss
- Cook for 15 minutes, divide between plates and serve.

24) KALE AND RAISINS

Preparation Time: 10 minutes   **Cooking Time:** 20 minutes   **Servings: 4**

Ingredients:
- 1 pound kale, torn
- 1 tomato, cubed
- 2 tablespoons avocado oil
- Juice of 1 lime
- ¼ cup raisins

Directions:
- Heat up a pan with the oil over medium heat

Ingredients:
- 1 teaspoon nutmeg, ground
- ½ teaspoon ginger, grated
- ½ teaspoon cinnamon powder
- 1 tablespoon chives, chopped
- A pinch of sea salt and black pepper

- Add the kale, tomato, lime juice and the other Ingredients, toss
- Cook for 20 minutes, divide into bowls and serve.

25) COLLARD GREENS AND GARLIC MIX

Preparation Time: 10 minutes   **Cooking Time**: 10 minutes   **Servings: 4**

Ingredients:
- 2 tablespoons avocado oil
- 4 garlic cloves, minced
- 4 bunches collard greens
- 1 tomato, cubed

Ingredients:
- A pinch of sea salt and black pepper
- Black pepper to the taste
- 1 tablespoon almonds, chopped

Directions:
- Heat up a pan with the oil over medium heat
- Add the garlic, collard greens
- Then the other ingredients, toss well
- Cook for 10 minutes, divide into bowls and serve.

26) CAULIFLOWER RICE AND CHIA MIX

Preparation Time: 10 minutes   **Cooking Time**: 15 minutes   **Servings: 4**

Ingredients:
- 2 cups cauliflower rice
- 2 tablespoons chia seeds
- ½ cup radishes, halved
- ½ cup chives, chopped

Ingredients:
- 2 tablespoons avocado oil
- Zest of 1 lime, grated
- 1 cup coconut cream

Directions:
- Heat up a pan with the oil over medium heat
- Add the cauliflower rice, chia seeds
- Add the other ingredients, toss
- Cook for 15 minutes, divide into bowls and serve.

27) FRUITY CAULIFLOWER RICE BOWLS

Preparation Time: 10 minutes   **Cooking Time**: 0 minutes   **Servings: 4**

Ingredients:
- ½ cup blackberries, halved
- ½ cup grapes, halved
- 2 cups cauliflower rice, steamed
- 1 cup cherry tomatoes, halved

Ingredients:
- 1 avocado, peeled, pitted and cubed
- 2 tablespoons avocado oil
- Juice of 1 lime

Directions:
- In a salad bowl, combine the cauliflower rice with the berries
- Add the other Ingredients, toss
- Divide into smaller bowls and serve.

28) SPICY ASIAN BROCCOLI

Preparation Time: 25 minutes   **Cooking Time**: 8 minutes   **Servings: 4**

Ingredients:
- 2 fresh limes' juice
- 2 small broccoli, cut into florets
- 2 teaspoon chili pepper, chopped

Ingredients:
- 2 tablespoons ginger, fresh, grated
- 4 garlic cloves, chopped
- 8 tablespoons olive oil

Directions:
- Add your broccoli florets into your steamer and steam them for 8 minutes.
- Meanwhile, to prepare dressing, add lime juice, garlic, chili pepper
- Then oil, and ginger in a small mixing bowl and combine
- Add steamed broccoli in a large mixing bowl
- Drizzle over it the dressing
- Toss to blend. Serve and enjoy!

29) TOMATO CUCUMBER CHEESE SALAD

Preparation Time: 15 minutes **Cooking Time:** As per dierections **Servings: 2**

Ingredients:
- 2 cups tomatoes, sliced
- 2 cucumbers, peeled, sliced
- 2 spring onions, sliced
- 7-ounces mozzarella cheese, chopped

Directions:
- In a large salad bowl, add basil pesto and cheese. Mix well

Ingredients:
- 12 black olives
- 2 teaspoons basil pesto
- 2 tablespoons extra-virgin olive oil
- 2 tablespoons basil, fresh, chopped
- Add remaining Ingredients into a bowl
- Toss to blend. Serve fresh and enjoy!

30) HEALTHY BRUSSELS SPROUT SALAD

Preparation Time: 15 minutes **Cooking Time:** As per dierections **Servings: 1**

Ingredients:
- ½ teaspoon apple cider vinegar
- 6 Brussels sprouts, washed, sliced
- 1 tablespoon Parmesan cheese, fresh, grated

Directions:
- Add all your Ingredients into a large salad bowl

Ingredients:
- 1 teaspoon extra-virgin olive oil
- ¼ teaspoon pepper
- ¼ teaspoon sea salt
- Toss to blend. Serve and enjoy!

31) HEALTHY BRAISED GARLIC KALE

Preparation Time: 50 minutes **Cooking Time:** As directions **Servings: 4**

Ingredients:
- 10 oz kale, stems removed and chopped
- 2 cups vegetable stock
- 4 tbsp coconut oil
- 1 tsp chili pepper flakes, dried

Directions:
- Heat coconut oil in a pan over medium heat.
- Once the oil is hot then add onion, garlic and chili pepper flakes
- Sauté until lightly brown. Pour vegetable stock and stir well.

Ingredients:
- 1 medium onion, sliced
- 4 garlic cloves, minced
- 1 tsp sea salt
- Now add chopped kale and season with salt. Stir well.
- Cover pan with lid and cook on low heat for 40 minutes.
- Serve and enjoy.

32) CAULIFLOWER LATKE

Preparation Time: 15 minutes **Cooking Time:** 30 minutes **Servings: 4**

Ingredients:
- 12 oz. cauliflower rice, cooked
- 1 egg, beaten
- 1/3 cup cornstarch

Directions:
- Squeeze excess water from the cauliflower rice using paper towels
- Place the cauliflower rice in a bowl.
- Stir in the egg and cornstarch
- Season with salt and pepper.
- Pour 2 tablespoons of oil into a pan over medium heat.

Ingredients:
- Salt and pepper to taste
- ¼ cup vegetable oil, divided
- Chopped onion chives
- Add 2 to 3 tablespoons of the cauliflower mixture into the pan
- Cook for 3 minutes per side or until golden.
- Repeat until you've used up the rest of the batter
- Garnish with chopped chives.

33) ROASTED BRUSSELS SPROUTS

Preparation Time: 30 minutes   **Cooking Time:** 20 minutes   **Servings: 4**

Ingredients:
- 1 lb. Brussels sprouts, sliced in half
- 1 shallot, chopped
- 1 tablespoon olive oil
- Salt and pepper to taste

Ingredients:
- 2 teaspoons balsamic vinegar
- ¼ cup pomegranate seeds
- ¼ cup goat cheese, crumbled

Directions:
- Preheat your oven to 400 degrees F
- Coat the Brussels sprouts with oil.
- Sprinkle with salt and pepper.
- Transfer to a baking pan.
- Roast in the oven for 20 minutes
- Drizzle with the vinegar.
- Sprinkle with the seeds and cheese before serving.

34) BRUSSELS SPROUTS & CRANBERRIES SALAD

Preparation Time: 10 minutes   **Cooking Time:** 0 minute   **Servings: 6**

Ingredients:
- 3 tablespoons lemon juice
- ¼ cup olive oil
- Salt and pepper to taste
- 1 lb. Brussels sprouts, sliced thinly

Ingredients:
- ¼ cup dried cranberries, chopped
- ½ cup pecans, toasted and chopped
- ½ cup vegan parmesan cheese, shaved

Directions:
- Mix the lemon juice, olive oil, salt and pepper in a bowl.
- Toss the Brussels sprouts, cranberries and pecans in this mixture
- Sprinkle the Parmesan cheese on top.

35) POTATO LATKE

Preparation Time: 15 minutes   **Cooking Time:** 10 minutes   **Servings: 6**

Ingredients:
- 3 eggs, beaten
- 1 onion, grated
- 1 ½ teaspoons baking powder
- Salt and pepper to taste

Ingredients:
- 2 lb. potatoes, peeled and grated
- ¼ cup all-purpose flour
- 4 tablespoons vegetable oil
- Chopped onion chives

Directions:
- Preheat your oven to 400 degrees F.
- In a bowl, beat the eggs, onion, baking powder, salt and pepper
- Squeeze moisture from the shredded potatoes using paper towel
- Add potatoes to the egg mixture.
- Stir in the flour. Pour the oil into a pan over medium heat.
- Cook a small amount of the batter for 3 to 4 minutes per side
- Repeat until the rest of the batter is used.
- Garnish with the chives.

36) BROCCOLI RABE

Preparation Time: 15 minutes **Cooking Time:** 15 minutes **Servings: 8**

Ingredients:
- 2.oranges, sliced in half
- 1 lb. broccoli rabe
- 1.tablespoons sesame oil, toasted

Directions:
- Pour the oil into a pan over medium heat
- Add the oranges and cook until caramelized
- Transfer to a plate.
- Put the broccoli in the pan
- Cook for 8 minutes

Ingredients:
- 1.Salt and pepper to taste
- 1 tablespoon sesame seeds, toasted

- Squeeze the oranges to release juice in a bowl.
- Stir in the oil, salt and pepper.
- Coat the broccoli rabe with the mixture
- Sprinkle seeds on top.

37) WHIPPED POTATOES

Preparation Time: 20 minutes **Cooking Time:** 35 minutes **Servings: 10**

Ingredients:
- 4 cups water
- 3 lb. potatoes, sliced into cubes
- 3 cloves garlic, crushed
- 6 tablespoons vegan butter
- 2 bay leaves

Directions:
- Boil the potatoes in water for 30 minutes or until tender. Drain.
- In a pan over medium heat, cook the garlic in butter for 1 minute
- Add the sage and cook for 5 more minutes.

Ingredients:
- 10 sage leaves
- ½ cup Vegan yogurt
- ¼ cup low-fat milk
- Salt to taste

- Discard the garlic. Use a fork to mash the potatoes.
- Whip using an electric mixer while gradually adding the butter, yogurt, and milk.
- Season with salt.

38) QUINOA AVOCADO SALAD

Preparation Time: 15 minutes **Cooking Time:** 4 minutes **Servings: 4**

Ingredients:
- 2 tablespoons balsamic vinegar
- ¼ cup cream
- ¼ cup buttermilk
- 5 tablespoons freshly squeezed lemon juice, divided
- 1 clove garlic, grated
- 2 tablespoons shallot, minced
- Salt and pepper to taste

Directions:
- Combine the vinegar, cream, milk, 1 tablespoon lemon juice
- Add garlic, shallot, salt and pepper in a bowl.
- Pour 1 tablespoon oil into a pan over medium heat
- Heat the quinoa for 4 minutes.
- Transfer quinoa to a plate.

Ingredients:
- 2 tablespoons avocado oil, divided
- 1 ¼ cups quinoa, cooked
- 2 heads endive, sliced
- 2 firm pears, sliced thinly
- 2 avocados, sliced
- ¼ cup fresh dill, chopped

- Toss the endive and pears in a mixture of remaining oil
- Add remaining lemon juice, salt and pepper.
- Transfer to a plate. Toss the avocado in the reserved dressing.
- Then to the plate. Top with the dill and quinoa.

39) ROASTED SWEET POTATOES

Preparation Time: 20 minutes **Cooking Time**: 20 minutes **Servings: 4**

Ingredients:
- 2 potatoes, sliced into wedges
- 2 tablespoons olive oil, divided
- Salt and pepper to taste
- 1 red bell pepper, chopped

Ingredients:
- ¼ cup fresh cilantro, chopped
- 1 garlic, minced
- 2 tablespoons almonds, toasted and sliced
- 1 tablespoon lime juice

Directions:
- Preheat your oven to 425 degrees F
- Toss the sweet potatoes in oil and salt
- Transfer to a baking pan.
- Roast for 20 minutes.
- In a bowl, combine the red bell pepper, cilantro, garlic and almonds
- In another bowl, mix the lime juice, remaining oil, salt and pepper
- Drizzle this mixture over the red bell pepper mixture.
- Serve sweet potatoes with the red bell pepper mixture.

40) CAULIFLOWER SALAD

Preparation Time: 20 minutes **Cooking Time**: 15 minutes **Servings: 4**

Ingredients:
- 8 cups cauliflower florets
- 5 tablespoons olive oil, divided
- Salt and pepper to taste
- 1 cup parsley
- 1 clove garlic, minced

Ingredients:
- 2 tablespoons lemon juice
- ¼ cup almonds, toasted and sliced
- 3 cups arugula
- 2 tablespoons olives, sliced
- ¼ cup feta, crumbled

Directions:
- Preheat your oven to 425 degrees F.
- Toss the cauliflower in a mixture of 1 tablespoon olive oil, salt and pepper
- Place in a baking pan and roast for 15 minutes.
- Put the parsley, remaining oil, garlic, lemon juice, salt and pepper in a blender.
- Pulse until smooth
- Place the roasted cauliflower in a salad bowl.
- Stir in the rest of the ingredients along with the parsley dressing.

SNACK RECIPES

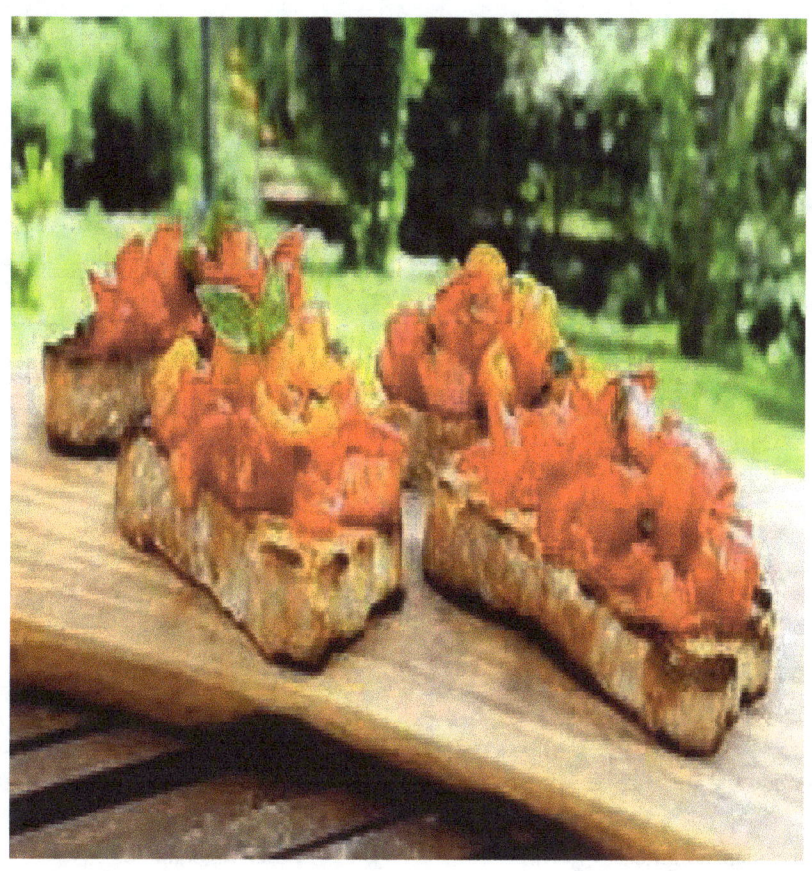

41) CANDIED ALMONDS

Preparation Time: 10 minutes   **Cooking Time:** 35 minutes   **Servings: 4**

Ingredients:
- 1 cup sugar
- 1/2 cup water

Ingredients:
- 2 cups whole almonds
- 1 tbsp cinnamon

Directions:
- In a pot over medium heat, boil water, cinnamon, and sugar
- Add almonds when water is boiling.
- Cook, stirring continuously, until liquid evaporates
- Place almonds on a towel in a single layer to drain. Let cool 15 minutes.
- Serve.

42) STUFFED MUSHROOMS

Preparation Time: 10 minutes   **Cooking Time:** 20 minutes   **Servings: 12**

Ingredients:
- 1 tbsp vegetable oil
- 12 whole fresh mushrooms
- 1 tbsp minced garlic
- 1/4 cup grated Parmesan

Ingredients:
- 8oz packaged softened cream cheese
- 1/4 tsp onion powder
- 1/4 tsp black pepper
- 1/4 tsp ground cayenne pepper

Directions:
- Preheat oven to 350 degrees Fahrenheit and spray a baking sheet with nonstick cooking spray.
- Wash mushrooms, pat dry, and break off stems. Chop stems very finely.
- In a large skillet over medium heat, cook garlic and mushroom stems in oil until moisture evaporates
- Then remove from heat. Stir in cream cheese after cooling; add black pepper, Parmesan
- Join also onion powder, and cayenne pepper until thick.
- Fill each mushroom cap with mixture and place caps on baking sheet
- Bake for 20 minutes. Serve warm.

43) KETTLE CORN

Preparation Time: 5 minutes   **Cooking Time:** 10 minutes   **Servings: 5**

Ingredients:
- 1/2 cup unpopped popcorn kernels
- 1/4 cup white sugar

Ingredients:
- 1/4 cup vegetable oil

Directions:
- Heat oil in a pot over medium heat until hot but not smoking
- Stir in popcorn and sugar.
- Cover and shake constantly while popcorn is popping.
- When popping slows to 3 seconds between pops, remove from heat
- Continue shaking for 2 minutes more.
- Pour into a bowl and let cool. Serve.

44) BLOOMING ONION

Preparation Time: 10 minutes   **Cooking Time:** 10 minutes   **Servings: 4**

Ingredients:
- 1 cup milk
- 1 egg
- 1 cup flour
- 1-1/2 tsp cayenne pepper
- 1-1/2 tsp salt
- 1 tsp paprika

Ingredients:
- 1/2 tsp black pepper
- 1/8 tsp thyme
- 1/3 tsp oregano
- 1/8 tsp cumin
- 3/4 cup vegetable oil
- 1 large onion

Directions:
- Beat egg and milk together in a large bowl.
- Combine salt, flour, cayenne pepper, black pepper, paprika
- Add thyme, oregano, and cumin in a separate bowl.
- Slice 1 inch from top and bottom of onion; peel off papery skin.
- Cut a 1 inch diameter core from the center of the onion with a thin knife.
- Slice 3/4 of the way through the onion with a sharp knife
- Then repeat in an X shape across the first slice. Continue until onion has been cut 12 to 16 times
- Do this carefully so as to not break the onion all the way through
- Spread onion petals apart. Dip onion into egg mixture, then coat well with flour mixture
- Dip into egg mixture again, then coat with flour mixture again
- Heat oil to 350 degrees Fahrenheit in a fryer or deep pot.
- Fry right side up for 10 minutes or until brown, then remove and let drain before serving.

45) BRUSCHETTA

Preparation Time: 10 minutes   **Cooking Time:** 5 minutes   **Servings: 4**

Ingredients:
- 1/2 cup grated Romano cheese
- 5 tbsp mayonnaise
- 1/3 cup chopped red onion

Ingredients:
- 6oz jar drained and chopped marinated artichoke hearts
- 1 French baguette, cut into 8 slices

Directions:
- Preheat oven broiler.
- Combine artichoke hearts with red onion, cheese, and mayonnaise in a large bowl,.
- Spread equal amounts of mixture over bread slices. Place slices on a baking sheet.
- Broil for 2 minutes. Serve warm.

46) SPICY JALAPEÑO POPPERS

Preparation Time: 10 minutes   **Cooking Time:** 30 minutes   **Servings: 12**

Ingredients:
- 8oz shredded sharp cheddar cheese
- 8oz softened cream cheese
- 15 seeded jalapeño peppers halved lengthwise

Ingredients:
- 1/4 cup mayonnaise
- 1/2 tbsp milk
- 2 beaten eggs
- 1-1/2 cups crushed corn flake cereal

Directions:
- Preheat oven to 350 degrees Fahrenheit; grease a baking sheet
- Combine cream cheese with mayonnaise and cheddar in a large bowl
- Stuff jalapeño halves with cheese mixture.
- In a separate bowl, whisk eggs together with milk.
- Dip jalapeños into egg mixture, then roll in corn flakes to coat well
- Bake on baking sheet in a single layer for 30 minutes. Serve.

47) MEXICAN ROLL-UPS

Preparation Time: 10 minutes **Cooking Time**: 0 minutes **Servings**: 8

Ingredients:
- 8oz cream cheese
- 2/3 cup chopped green olives
- 1/3 cup mayonnaise
- 2 oz canned chopped black olives

Ingredients:
- 1/2 cup salsa
- 6 chopped green onions
- 8 flour tortillas

Directions:
- Combine cream cheese in a large bowl with green olives
- Add mayonnaise, black olives, and green onions.
- Thinly spread cream cheese mixture onto tortillas
- Roll up tightly and chill for 1 hour.
- Slice into pieces and serve topped with salsa.

48) BAKED ZUCCHINI

Preparation Time: 10 minutes **Cooking Time**: 10 minutes **Servings**: 4

Ingredients:
- 1/2 cup Italian bread crumbs
- 2 thinly sliced zucchinis
- 1/8 tsp black pepper

Ingredients:
- 2 tbsp grated Parmesan
- 2 egg whites

Directions:
- Preheat oven to 475 degrees Fahrenheit.
- Stir bread crumbs together with Parmesan and pepper in a small bowl
- Place egg whites in a separate small bowl.
- Dip zucchini slices into egg whites, then breadcrumb mixture
- Arrange in a single layer on a baking sheet.
- Bake for 5 minutes, flip, and bake for 5 more minutes. Serve.

49) PUMPKIN SEEDS

Preparation Time: 10 minutes **Cooking Time**: 1hour **Servings**: 4

Ingredients:
- 1/2 tsp salt
- 1-1/2 tbsp melted margarine
- 1/8 tsp garlic salt

Ingredients:
- 2 cups raw pumpkin seeds
- 2 tsp Worcestershire sauce

Directions:
- Preheat oven to 275 degrees Fahrenheit.
- In a large bowl, combine garlic salt, margarine, salt, and Worcestershire sauce.
- Stir pumpkin seeds into mixture. Place on a baking sheet.
- Bake for 1 hour, stirring a few times throughout. Let cool. Serve.

50) SPINACH BARS

Preparation Time: 10 minutes **Cooking Time:** 40 minutes **Servings: 12**

Ingredients:
- 1 cup flour
- 1 tsp baking powder
- 1 tsp salt
- 10oz rinsed and chopped fresh spinach
- 2 eggs

Ingredients:
- 1/2 cup melted butter
- 1 cup milk
- 1 chopped onion
- 8 oz shredded mozzarella cheese

Directions:
- Preheat oven to 375 degrees Fahrenheit and grease a baking dish.
- Boil spinach in a pot on the stove over medium-high heat
- When boiling, lower temperature to low
- Simmer for 3 minutes or until spinach is wilted. Drain spinach.
- Combine flour, baking powder, and salt in a large bowl
- Then stir in butter, eggs, milk, onion, spinach, and mozzarella.
- Place mixture in baking dish and spread evenly
- Bake for 35 minutes.
- Let cool, then slice into bars. Serve.

51) QUINOA BROCCOLI TOTS

Preparation Time: 10 minutes **Cooking Time:** 20 minutes **Servings: 16**

Ingredients:
- 2 tablespoons quinoa flour
- 2 cups steamed and chopped broccoli florets
- 1/2 cup nutritional yeast
- 1 teaspoon garlic powder

Ingredients:
- 1 teaspoon miso paste
- 2 flax eggs
- 2 tablespoons hummus

Directions:
- Place all the ingredients in a bowl, stir until well combined
- Then shape the mixture into sixteen small balls.
- Arrange the balls on a baking sheet lined with parchment paper
- Spray with oil and bake at 400 degrees F for 20 minutes until brown, turning halfway.
- When done, let the tots cool for 10 minutes. Serve straight away

52) SPICY ROASTED CHICKPEAS

Preparation Time: 10 minutes **Cooking Time:** 20 minutes **Servings: 6**

Ingredients:
- 30 ounces cooked chickpeas
- ½ teaspoon salt
- 2 teaspoons mustard powder

Ingredients:
- ½ teaspoon cayenne pepper
- 2 tablespoons olive oil

Directions:
- Place all the ingredients in a bowl and stir until well coated
- Then spread the chickpeas in an even layer on a baking sheet greased with oil.
- Bake the chickpeas for 20 minutes at 400 degrees F until golden brown and crispy
- Serve straight away.

53) NACHO KALE CHIPS

Preparation Time: 10 minutes   **Cooking Time**: 14 hours   **Servings**: 10

Ingredients:
- 2 bunches of curly kale
- 2 cups cashews, soaked, drained
- 1/2 cup chopped red bell pepper
- 1 teaspoon garlic powder
- 1 teaspoon salt
- 2 tablespoons red chili powder

Ingredients:
- 1/2 teaspoon smoked paprika
- 1/2 cup nutritional yeast
- 1 teaspoon cayenne
- 3 tablespoons lemon juice
- 3/4 cup water

Directions:
- Place all the ingredients except for kale in a food processor and pulse for 2 minutes until smooth.
- Place kale in a large bowl, pour in the blended mixture
- Mix until coated, and dehydrate for 14 hours at 120 degrees F until crispy.
- If dehydrator is not available, spread kale between two baking sheets
- Bake for 90 minutes at 225 degrees F until crispy, flipping halfway.
- When done, let chips cool for 15 minutes and then serve

54) RED SALSA

Preparation Time: 10 minutes   **Cooking Time**: 0 minute   **Servings**: 8

Ingredients:
- 30 ounces diced fire-roasted tomatoes
- 4 tablespoons diced green chilies
- 1 medium jalapeño pepper, deseeded
- 1/2 cup chopped green onion
- 1 cup chopped cilantro

Ingredients:
- 1 teaspoon minced garlic
- ½ teaspoon of sea salt
- 1 teaspoon ground cumin
- ¼ teaspoon stevia
- 3 tablespoons lime juice

Directions:
- Place all the ingredients in a food processor and process for 2 minutes until smooth.
- Tip the salsa in a bowl, taste to adjust seasoning and then serve.

55) TOMATO HUMMUS

Preparation Time: 5 minutes   **Cooking Time**: 0 minute   **Servings**: 4

Ingredients:
- 1/4 cup sun-dried tomatoes, without oil
- 1 ½ cups cooked chickpeas
- 1 teaspoon minced garlic
- 1/2 teaspoon salt

Ingredients:
- 2 tablespoons sesame oil
- 1 tablespoon lemon juice
- 1 tablespoon olive oil
- 1/4 cup of water

Directions:
- Place all the ingredients in a food processor
- Process for 2 minutes until smooth.
- Tip the hummus in a bowl
- Drizzle with more oil, and then serve straight away.

56) MARINATED MUSHROOMS

Preparation Time: 10 minutes **Cooking Time:** 7 minutes **Servings: 6**

Ingredients:
- 12 ounces small button mushrooms
- 1 teaspoon minced garlic
- 1/4 teaspoon dried thyme
- 1/2 teaspoon sea salt
- 1/2 teaspoon dried basil
- 1/2 teaspoon red pepper flakes

Directions:
- Take a skillet pan, place it over medium-high heat
- Add 1 teaspoon oil and when hot, add mushrooms
- Cook for 5 minutes until golden brown.

Ingredients:
- 1/4 teaspoon dried oregano
- 1/2 teaspoon maple syrup
- 1/4 cup apple cider vinegar
- 1/4 cup and 1 teaspoon olive oil
- 2 tablespoons chopped parsley

- Meanwhile, prepare the marinade and for this, place remaining ingredients in a bowl
- Whisk until combined. When mushrooms have cooked, transfer them into the bowl of marinade
- Toss until well coated. Serve straight away

57) HUMMUS QUESADILLAS

Preparation Time: 5 minutes **Cooking Time:** 15 minutes **Servings: 1**

Ingredients:
- 1 tortilla, whole wheat
- 1/4 cup diced roasted red peppers
- 1 cup baby spinach
- 1/3 teaspoon minced garlic
- ¼ teaspoon salt

Directions:
- Place a large pan over medium heat
- Add oil and when hot, add red peppers and garlic
- Season with salt and black pepper and cook for 3 minutes until sauté.
- Then stir in spinach, cook for 1 minute
- Remove the pan from heat and transfer the mixture in a bowl.

Ingredients:
- ¼ teaspoon ground black pepper
- 1/4 teaspoon olive oil
- 1/4 cup hummus
- Oil as needed

- Prepare quesadilla and for this, spread hummus on one-half of the tortilla
- Then spread spinach mixture on it, cover the filling with the other half of the tortilla
- Cook in a pan for 3 minutes per side until browned.
- When done, cut the quesadilla into wedges and serve

58) NACHO CHEESE SAUCE

Preparation Time: 5 minutes **Cooking Time:** 10 minutes **Servings: 4**

Ingredients:
- 3 tablespoons flour
- 1/4 teaspoon garlic salt
- 1/4 teaspoon salt
- 1/2 teaspoon cumin
- 1/4 teaspoon paprika

Directions:
- Take a small saucepan, place it over medium heat
- Pour in vegetable broth, and bring it to a boil.
- Then whisk together flour and yogurt, add to the boiling broth

Ingredients:
- 1 teaspoon red chili powder
- 1/8 teaspoon cayenne powder
- 1 cup vegan cashew yogurt
- 1 1/4 cups vegetable broth

- Stir in all the spices, switch heat to medium-low level
- Cook for 5 minutes until thickened. Serve straight away.

59) **AVOCADO TOMATO BRUSCHETTA**

Preparation Time: 10 minutes   **Cooking Time:** 0 minute   **Servings: 4**

Ingredients:
- 3 slices of whole-grain bread
- 6 chopped cherry tomatoes
- ½ of sliced avocado
- ½ teaspoon minced garlic

Ingredients:
- ½ teaspoon ground black pepper
- 2 tablespoons chopped basil
- ½ teaspoon of sea salt
- 1 teaspoon balsamic vinegar

Directions:
- Place tomatoes in a bowl, and then stir in vinegar until mixed.
- Top bread slices with avocado slices
- Then top evenly with tomato mixture, garlic and basil
- Season with salt and black pepper. Serve straight away

60) **CINNAMON BANANAS**

Preparation Time: 5 minutes   **Cooking Time:** 8 minutes   **Servings: 2**

Ingredients:
- 2 bananas, peeled, sliced
- 1 teaspoon cinnamon

Ingredients:
- 2 tablespoons granulated Splenda
- 1/4 teaspoon nutmeg

Directions:
- Prepare the cinnamon mixture and for this, place all the ingredients in a bowl, except for banana
- Stir until mixed. Take a large skillet pan, place it over medium heat
- Spray with oil, add banana slices and sprinkle with half of the prepared cinnamon mixture.
- Cook for 3 minutes, then sprinkle with remaining prepared cinnamon mixture
- Continue to cook for 3 minutes until tender and hot. Serve straight away

DINNER RECIPES

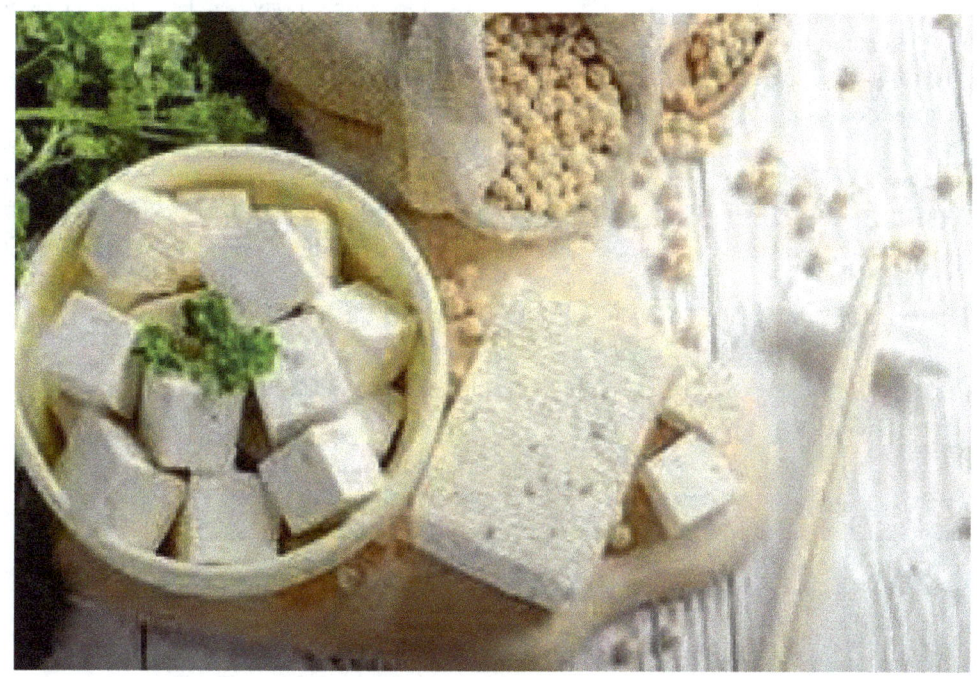

61) GINGER LIME TEMPEH

Preparation Time: 10 minutes **Cooking Time:** 40 minutes **Servings: 4**

Ingredients:
- 5 kaffir lime leaves
- 1 tbsp cumin powder
- 1 tbsp ginger powder
- 1 cup plain unsweetened yogurt

Directions:
- In a large bowl, combine the kaffir lime leaves, cumin, ginger, and plain yogurt
- Add the tempeh, season with salt, and black pepper, and mix to coat well
- Cover the bowl with a plastic wrap and marinate in the refrigerator for 2 to 3 hours.
- Preheat the oven to 350 f and grease a baking sheet with cooking spray.
- Take out the tempeh and arrange on the baking sheet

Ingredients:
- 2 lb tempeh
- Salt and ground black pepper to taste
- 1 tbsp olive oil
- 1 limes, juiced

- Drizzle with olive oil, lime juice, cover with aluminum foil
- Slow-cook in the oven for 1 to 1 ½ hours or until the tempeh cooks within.
- Remove the aluminum foil, turn the broiler side of the oven on
- Brown the top of the tempeh for 5 to 10 minutes.
- Take out the tempeh and serve warm with red cabbage slaw.

62) TOFU MOZZARELLA

Preparation Time: 10minutes **Cooking Time:** 35minutes **Servings: 4**

Ingredients:
- 1½ lb tofu, halved lengthwise
- Salt and ground black pepper to taste
- 2 eggs
- 2 tbsp italian seasoning
- 1 pinch red chili flakes
- ½ cup sliced pecorino romano cheese
- ¼ cup fresh parsley, chopped

Directions:
- Preheat the oven to 400 f and grease a baking dish with cooking spray. Set aside.
- Season the tofu with salt and black pepper; set aside.
- In a medium bowl, whisk the eggs with the italian seasoning, and red chili flakes
- In a plate, combine the pecorino romano cheese with parsley.
- Melt the butter in a medium skillet over medium heat.
- Quickly dip the tofu in the egg mixture and then dredge generously in the cheese mixture
- Place in the butter and fry on both sides
- (Until the cheese melts and is golden brown, 8 to 10 minutes)

Ingredients:
- 4 tbsp butter
- 2 garlic cloves, minced
- 2 cups crushed tomatoes
- 1 tbsp dried basil
- Salt and ground black pepper to taste
- ½ lb sliced mozzarella cheese

- Place on a plate and set aside.
- Sauté the garlic in the same pan and mix in the tomatoes
- Top with the basil, salt, and black pepper
- Cook for 5 to 10 minutes. Pour the sauce into the baking dish.
- Lay the tofu pieces in the sauce and top with the mozzarella cheese
- Bake in the oven for 10 to 15 minutes or until the cheese melts completely.
- Remove the dish and serve with leafy green salad.

63) SEITAN MEATZA WITH KALE

Preparation Time: 10 minutes **Cooking Time:** 22 minutes **Servings: 4**

Ingredients:
- 1 lb ground seitan
- Salt and black pepper to taste
- 2 cups powdered parmesan cheese
- ¼ tsp onion powder
- ¼ tsp garlic powder

Ingredients:
- ½ cup unsweetened tomato sauce
- 1 tsp white vinegar
- ½ tsp liquid smoke
- ¼ cup baby kale, chopped roughly
- 1 cup mozzarella cheese

Directions:
- Preheat the oven to 400 f and line a medium pizza pan with parchment paper
- Grease with cooking spray. Set aside.
- In a medium bowl, combine the seitan, salt, black pepper, and parmesan cheese
- Spread the mixture on the pizza pan to fit the shape of the pan
- Bake in the oven for 15 minutes or until the meat cooks.
- Meanwhile in a medium bowl, mix the onion powder, garlic powder
- Add tomato sauce, vinegar, and liquid smoke.
- Remove the meat crust from the oven and spread the tomato mixture on top
- Add the kale and sprinkle with the mozzarella cheese.
- Bake in the oven for 7 minutes or until the cheese melts.
- Take out from the oven, slice, and serve warm.

64) TACO TEMPEH CASSEROLE

Preparation Time: 10 minutes **Cooking Time:** 20 minutes **Servings: 4**

Ingredients:
- 1 tempeh, shredded
- 1/3 cup vegan mayonnaise
- 8 oz dairy- free cream cheese (vegan 1 yellow onion, sliced
- 1 yellow bell pepper, deseeded and chopped

Ingredients:
- 2 tbsp taco seasoning
- ½ cup shredded cheddar cheese
- Salt and ground black pepper to taste

Directions:
- Preheat the oven to 400 f and grease a baking dish with cooking spray.
- Into the dish, put the tempeh, mayonnaise, cashew cream, onion
- Then bell pepper, taco seasoning, and two-thirds of the cheese, salt, and black pepper
- Mix the ingredients and top with the remaining cheese.
- Bake in the oven for 15 to 20 minutes or until the cheese melts and is golden brown.
- Remove the dish, plate, and serve with lettuce leaves

65) BROCCOLI TEMPEH ALFREDO

Preparation Time: 10minutes **Cooking Time:** 15minutes **Servings: 4**

Ingredients:
- 6 slices tempeh, chopped
- 2 tbsp butter
- 4 tofu, cut into 1-inch cubes
- Salt and ground black pepper to taste
- 4 garlic cloves, minced

Ingredients:
- 1 cup baby kale, chopped
- 1 ½ cups full- fat heavy cream
- 1 medium head broccoli, cut into florets
- ¼ cup shredded parmesan cheese directions:

Directions:
- Put the tempeh in a medium skillet over medium heat and fry until crispy and brown, 5 minutes.
- Spoon onto a plate and set aside. Melt the butter in the same skillet
- Season the tofu with salt and black pepper, and cook on both sides until golden brown
- Spoon onto the tempeh's plate and set aside.
- Add the garlic to the skillet, sauté for 1 minute.
- Mix in the full- fat heavy cream, tofu, and tempeh, and kale
- Allow simmering for 5 minutes or until the sauce thickens.
- Meanwhile, pour the broccoli into a large safe- microwave bowl
- Sprinkle with some water, season with salt, and black pepper
- Microwave for 2 minutes or until the broccoli softens.
- Spoon the broccoli into the sauce, top with the parmesan cheese
- Stir and cook until the cheese melts. Turn the heat off.
- Spoon the mixture into a serving platter and serve warm

66) AVOCADO SEITAN

Preparation Time: 10 minutes **Cooking Time:** 2 hours 15 minutes **Servings: 4**

Ingredients:
- 1 white onion, finely chopped
- ¼ cup vegetable stock
- 3 tbsp coconut oil
- 3 tbsp tamari sauce
- 3 tbsp chili pepper

Directions:
- In a large pot, combine the onion, vegetable stock, coconut oil
- Then tamari sauce, chili pepper, red wine vinegar, salt, black pepper
- Add the seitan, close the lid, and cook over low heat for 2 hours.

Ingredients:
- 1 tbsp red wine vinegar
- Salt and ground black pepper to taste
- 2 lb seitan
- 1 large avocado, halved and pitted
- ½ lemon, juiced
- Scoop the avocado pulp into a bowl, add the lemon juice, and using a fork
- Mash the avocado into a puree. Set aside.
- When ready, turn the heat off and mix in the avocado
- Adjust the taste with salt and black pepper.
- Spoon onto a serving platter and serve warm

67) SEITAN MUSHROOM BURGERS

Preparation Time: 15 minutes **Cooking Time:** 13 minutes **Servings: 4**

Ingredients:
- 1 ½ lb ground seitan
- Salt and ground black pepper to taste 1 tbsp unsweetened tomato sauce
- 6 large portobello caps, destemmed 1 tbsp olive oil
- 6 slices cheddar cheese for topping:

Directions:
- In a medium bowl, combine the seitan, salt, black pepper, and tomato sauce
- Use your hands, mold the mixture into 4 patties, and set aside.
- Rinse the mushrooms under running water and pat dry.
- Heat the olive oil in a medium skillet
- Place in the portobello caps and cook until softened, 3 to 4 minutes
- Transfer to a serving plate and set aside.

Ingredients:
- 4 lettuce leaves
- 4 large tomato slices
- ¼ cup mayonnaise

- Put the seitan patties in the skillet and fry on both sides (
- Until brown and compacted, 8 minutes)
- Place the vegan cheddar slices on the food
- Allow melting for 1 minute and lift each patty onto each mushroom cap.
- Divide the lettuce on top, then the tomato slices,
- Add some mayonnaise. Serve immediately.

68) TACO TEMPEH STUFFED PEPPERS

Preparation Time: 15 minutes **Cooking Time:** 41 minutes **Servings: 6**

Ingredients:
- 6 yellow bell peppers, halved and deseeded
- 1 ½ tbsp olive oil
- Salt and ground black pepper to taste
- 3 tbsp butter
- 3 garlic cloves, minced

Directions:
- Preheat the oven to 400 f and grease a baking dish with cooking spray. Set aside.
- Drizzle the bell peppers with the olive oil and season with some salt. Set aside.
- Melt the butter in a large skillet and sauté the garlic and onion for 3 minutes
- Stir in the tempeh, taco seasoning, salt, and black pepper
- Cook until the meat is no longer pink, 8 minutes.
- Mix in the broccoli until adequately incorporated. Turn the heat off.

Ingredients:
- ½ white onion, chopped
- 2 lbs. Ground tempeh
- 3 tsp taco seasoning
- 1 cup riced broccoli
- ¼ cup grated cheddar cheese
- Plain unsweetened yogurt for serving

- Spoon the mixture into the peppers, top with the cheddar cheese
- Place the peppers in the baking dish
- Bake in the oven until the cheese melts and is bubbly, 30 minutes.
- Remove the dish from the oven and plate the peppers
- Top with the palin yogurt and serve warm.

69) TANGY TOFU MEATLOAF

Preparation Time: 10 minutes   **Cooking Time:** 40 minutes   **Servings: 6**

Ingredients:
- 2 ½ lb ground tofu
- Salt and ground black pepper to taste
- 3 tbsp flaxseed meal
- 2 large eggs
- 2 tbsp olive oil

Ingredients:
- 1 lemon,1 tbsp juiced
- ¼ cup freshly chopped parsley
- ¼ cup freshly chopped oregano
- 4 garlic cloves, minced
- Lemon slices to garnish

Directions:
- Preheat the oven to 400 f and grease a loaf pan with cooking spray. Set aside.
- In a large bowl, combine the tofu, salt, black pepper, and flaxseed meal. Set aside.
- In a small bowl, whisk the eggs with the olive oil, lemon juice, parsley, oregano, and garlic.
- our the mixture onto the mix and combine well.
- Spoon the tofu mixture into the loaf pan and press to fit into the pan
- Bake in the middle rack of the oven for 30 to 40 minutes.
- Remove the pan, tilt to drain the meat's liquid, and allow cooling for 5 minutes.
- Slice, garnish with some lemon slices and serve with braised green beans.

70) VEGAN BACON WRAPPED TOFU WITH BUTTERED SPINACH

Preparation Time: 5 minutes   **Cooking Time:** 20 minutes   **Servings: 4**

Ingredients:
- For the bacon wrapped tofu:
- 4 tofu
- 8 slices vegan bacon
- Salt and black pepper to taste
- 2 tbsp olive oil

Ingredients:
- For the buttered spinach:
- 2 tbsp butter
- 1 lb spinach
- 4 garlic cloves
- Salt and ground black pepper to taste

Directions:
- For the bacon wrapped tofu:
- Preheat the oven to 450 f.
- Wrap each tofu with two vegan bacon slices
- Season with salt and black pepper, and place on the baking sheet
- Drizzle with the olive oil and bake in the oven for 15 minutes
- (Or until the vegan bacon browns and the tofu cooks within)
- For the buttered spinach:
- Meanwhile, melt the butter in a large skillet
- Add and sauté the spinach and garlic until the leaves wilt, 5 minutes
- Season with salt and black pepper.
- Remove the tofu from the oven and serve with the buttered spinach.

71) CAULIFLOWER MIX

Preparation Time: 10 minutes   **Cooking Time:** 25 minutes   **Servings: 4**

Ingredients:
- 1 pound cauliflower florets
- 2 tablespoons avocado oil
- 1 teaspoon nutmeg, ground
- 1 teaspoon hot paprika

Ingredients:
- 1 tablespoon pumpkin seeds
- 1 tablespoon chives, chopped
- A pinch of sea salt and black pepper

Directions:
- Spread the cauliflower florets on a baking sheet lined with parchment paper
- Add the oil, the nutmeg and the other ingredients, toss
- Bake at 380 degrees F for 25 minutes.
- Divide the cauliflower mix between plates and serve.

72) BAKED BROCCOLI AND PINE NUTS

Preparation Time: 10 minutes   **Cooking Time:** 30 minutes   **Servings: 4**

Ingredients:
- 2 tablespoons olive oil
- 1 pound broccoli florets
- 1 tablespoon garlic, minced
- 1 tablespoon pine nuts, toasted

Ingredients:
- 1 tablespoon lemon juice
- 2 teaspoons mustard
- A pinch of salt and black pepper

Directions:
- In a roasting pan, combine the broccoli with the oil, the garlic
- Add the other ingredients, toss
- Bake at 380 degrees F for 30 minutes.
- Divide everything between plates and serve.

73) CHILI ASPARAGUS

Preparation Time: 10 minutes   **Cooking Time:** 15 minutes   **Servings: 4**

Ingredients:
- 1 yellow onion, chopped
- 2 tablespoons olive oil
- 1 bunch asparagus, trimmed and halved

Ingredients:
- 2 garlic cloves, minced
- 1 teaspoon chili powder
- ¼ cup cilantro, chopped

Directions:
- Heat up a pan with the oil over medium-high heat
- Add the onion and the garlic and sauté for 5 minutes.
- Then the asparagus and the other ingredients, toss
- Cook for 10 minutes, divide between plates and serve.

74) TOMATO QUINOA

Preparation Time: 10 minutes   **Cooking Time:** 25 minutes   **Servings: 4**

Ingredients:
- 1 cup quinoa
- 3 cups chicken stock
- 1 cup tomatoes, cubed
- 1 tablespoon parsley, chopped

Ingredients:
- 1 tablespoon basil, chopped
- 1 teaspoon turmeric powder
- A pinch of salt and black pepper

Directions:
- In a pot, mix the quinoa with the stock, the tomatoes
- Add the other ingredients, toss
- Bring to a simmer and cook over medium heat for 25 minutes.
- Divide everything between plates and serve.

75) CORIANDER BLACK BEANS

Preparation Time: 10 minutes   **Cooking Time:** 20 minutes   **Servings: 4**

Ingredients:
- 1 tablespoon olive oil
- 2 cups canned black beans, drained and rinsed
- 1 green bell pepper, chopped
- 1 yellow onion, chopped
- 4 garlic cloves, minced

Ingredients:
- 1 teaspoon cumin, ground
- ½ cup chicken stock
- 1 tablespoon coriander, chopped
- A pinch of salt and black pepper

Directions:
- Heat up a pan with the oil over medium heat
- Add the onion and the garlic and sauté for 5 minutes.
- Then the black beans and the other ingredients, toss
- Cook over medium heat for 15 minutes more
- Divide between plates and serve.

76) **GREEN BEANS AND MANGO MIX**

Preparation Time: 10 minutes   **Cooking Time**: 20 minutes   **Servings: 4**

Ingredients:
- 1 pound green beans, trimmed and halved
- 3 scallions, chopped
- 1 mango, peeled and cubed
- 2 tablespoons olive oil

Directions:
- Heat up a pan with the oil over medium heat
- Add the scallions and sauté for 2 minutes.

Ingredients:
- ½ cup veggie stock
- 1 tablespoon oregano, chopped
- 1 teaspoon sweet paprika
- A pinch of salt and black pepper
- Then the green beans and the other ingredients, toss
- Cook over medium heat for 18 minutes more
- Divide between plates and serve.

77) **QUINOA WITH OLIVES**

Preparation Time: 10 minutes   **Cooking Time**: 30 minutes   **Servings: 4**

Ingredients:
- 1 yellow onion, chopped
- 1 tablespoon olive oil
- 1 cup quinoa
- 3 cups vegetable stock
- ½ cup black olives, pitted and halved

Directions:
- Heat up a pot with the oil over medium heat
- Add the yellow onion and sauté for 5 minutes.
- Then the quinoa and the other ingredients except the green onions, stir

Ingredients:
- 2 green onions, chopped
- 2 tablespoons coconut aminos
- 1 teaspoon rosemary, dried

- Bring to a simmer and cook over medium heat for 25 minutes.
- Divide the mix between plates
- Sprinkle the green onions on top and serve.

78) **GARLIC ASPARAGUS AND TOMATOES**

Preparation Time: 10 minutes   **Cooking Time**: 20 minutes   **Servings: 4**

Ingredients:
- 1 pound asparagus, trimmed and halved
- ½ pound cherry tomatoes, halved
- 2 tablespoons olive oil
- 1 teaspoon turmeric powder

Directions:
- Spread the asparagus on a baking sheet lined with parchment paper
- Add the tomatoes and the other ingredients, toss

Ingredients:
- 2 tablespoons shallot, chopped
- A pinch of salt and black pepper
- 1 tablespoon chives, chopped

- Cook in the oven at 375 degrees F for 20 minutes.
- Divide everything between plates and serve

79) HOT CUCUMBER MIX

Preparation Time: 10 minutes **Cooking Time**: 0 minutes **Servings**: 4

Ingredients:
- 1 pound cucumbers, sliced
- 1 tablespoon olive oil
- 1 teaspoon chili powder
- 1 green chili, chopped

Ingredients:
- 1 garlic clove, minced
- 1 tablespoon dill, chopped
- 2 tablespoons lime juice
- 1 tablespoon balsamic vinegar

Directions:
- In a bowl, combine the cucumbers with the garlic, the oil
- Add the other ingredients
- Toss and serve as a salad.

80) TOMATO SALAD

Preparation Time: 10 minutes **Cooking Time**: 0 minutes **Servings**: 4

Ingredients:
- 1 pound cherry tomatoes, halved
- 3 scallions, chopped
- 1 tablespoon olive oil

Ingredients:
- A pinch of salt and black pepper
- 1 tablespoon lime juice
- ¼ cup parsley, chopped

Directions:
- In a bowl, combine the tomatoes with the scallions
- Add the other ingredients
- Toss and serve as a salad.

DESSERT RECIPES

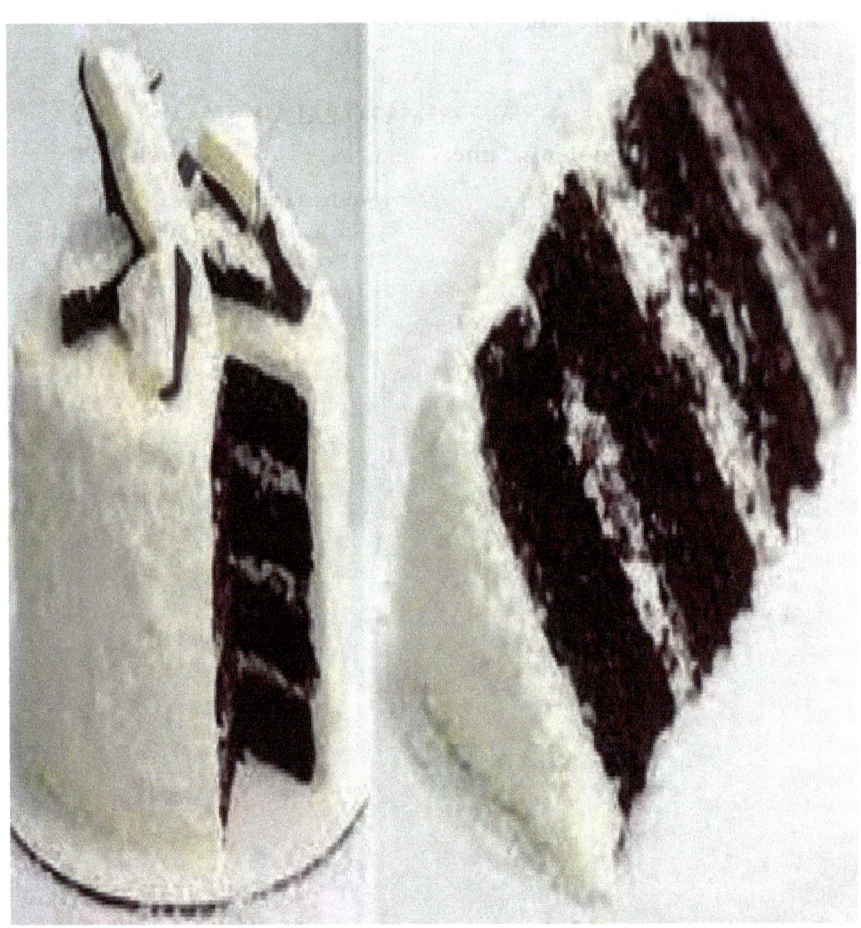

81) CHOCOLATE WATERMELON CUPS

Preparation Time: 2 hours   **Cooking Time**: 0 minutes   **Servings**: 4

Ingredients:
- 2 cups watermelon, peeled and cubed
- 1 tablespoon stevia
- 1 cup coconut cream

Ingredients:
- 1 tablespoon cocoa powder
- 1 tablespoon mint, chopped

Directions:
- In a blender, combine the watermelon with the stevia
- Add the other ingredients
- Pulse well, divide into cups
- Keep in the fridge for 2 hours before serving.

82) VANILLA RASPBERRIES MIX

Preparation Time: 10 minutes   **Cooking Time**: 10 minutes   **Servings**: 4

Ingredients:
- 1 cup water
- 1 cup raspberries
- 3 tablespoons stevia

Ingredients:
- 1 teaspoon nutmeg, ground
- ½ teaspoon vanilla extract

Directions:
- In a pan, combine the raspberries with the water
- Add the other ingredients
- Toss, cook over medium heat for 10 minutes
- Divide into bowls and serve.

83) COCONUT SALAD

Preparation Time: 10 minutes   **Cooking Time**: 0 minutes   **Servings**: 6

Ingredients:
- 2 cups coconut flesh, unsweetened and shredded
- ½ cup walnuts, chopped
- 1 cup blackberries

Ingredients:
- 1 tablespoon stevia
- 1 tablespoon coconut oil, melted

Directions:
- In a bowl, combine the coconut with the walnuts
- Add the other ingredients:, toss and serve.

84) MINT COOKIES

Preparation Time: 10 minutes   **Cooking Time**: 20 minutes   **Servings**: 6

Ingredients:
- 2 cups coconut flour
- 3 tablespoons flaxseed mixed with
- 4 tablespoons water
- ½ cup coconut cream

Ingredients:
- ½ cup coconut oil, melted
- 3 tablespoons stevia
- 2 teaspoons mint, dried
- 2 teaspoons baking soda

Directions:
- In a bowl, mix the coconut flour with the flaxseed, coconut cream
- Add the other ingredients, and whisk really well.
- Shape balls out of this mix, place them on a lined baking sheet, flatten them
- Introduce in the oven at 370 degrees F
- Bake for 20 minutes. Serve the cookies cold.

85) MINT AVOCADO BARS

Preparation Time: 10 minutes **Cooking Time:** 25 minutes **Servings: 6**

Ingredients:
- 1 teaspoon almond extract
- ½ cup coconut oil, melted
- 2 tablespoons stevia

Directions:
- In a bowl, combine the coconut oil with the almond extract
- Add stevia and the other ingredients and whisk well.

Ingredients:
- 1 avocado, peeled, pitted and mashed
- 2 cups coconut flour
- 1 tablespoon cocoa powder

- Transfer this to baking pan, spread evenly
- Introduce in the oven and cook at 370 degrees F
- Bake for 25 minutes. Cool down, cut into bars and serve.

86) COCONUT CHOCOLATE CAKE

Preparation Time: 10 minutes **Cooking Time:** 30 minutes **Servings: 12**

Ingredients:
- 4 tablespoons flaxseed mixed with
- 5 tablespoons water
- 1 cup coconut flesh, unsweetened and shredded
- 1 teaspoon vanilla extract
- 2 tablespoons cocoa powder

Directions:
- In a bowl, combine the flaxmeal with the coconut, the vanilla
- Add the other Ingredients

Ingredients:
- 1 teaspoon baking soda
- 2 cups almond flour
- 4 tablespoons stevia
- 2 tablespoons lime zest
- 2 cups coconut cream

- Whisk well and transfer to a cake pan.
- Cook the cake at 360 degree F for 30 minutes
- Cool down and serve.

87) MINT CHOCOLATE CREAM

Preparation Time: 10 minutes **Cooking Time:** 0 minutes **Servings: 6**

Ingredients:
- 1 cup coconut oil, melted
- 4 tablespoons cocoa powder
- 1 teaspoon vanilla extract

Directions:
- In your food processor, combine the coconut oil with the cocoa powder

Ingredients:
- 1 cup mint, chopped
- 2 cups coconut cream
- 4 tablespoons stevia

- Add the cream and the other ingredients, pulse well
- Divide into bowls and serve really cold.

88) CRANBERRIES CAKE

Preparation Time: 10 minutes **Cooking Time:** 30 minutes **Servings: 6**

Ingredients:
- 2 cups coconut flour
- 2 tablespoon coconut oil, melted
- 3 tablespoons stevia
- 1 tablespoon cocoa powder, unsweetened
- 2 tablespoons flaxseed mixed with

Directions:
- In a bowl, combine the coconut flour with the coconut oil
- Add the stevia and the other ingredients, and whisk well.
- Pour this into a cake pan lined with parchment paper

Ingredients:
- 3 tablespoons water
- 1 cup cranberries
- 1 cup coconut cream
- ¼ teaspoon vanilla extract
- ½ teaspoon baking powder
- Introduce in the oven
- Cook at 360 degrees F for 30 minutes.
- Cool down, slice and serve.

89) SWEET ZUCCHINI BUNS

Preparation Time: 10 minutes **Cooking Time:** As per directions **Servings: 8**

Ingredients:
- 1 cup almond flour
- 1/3 cup coconut flesh, unsweetened and shredded
- 1 cup zucchinis, grated
- 2 tablespoons stevia
- 1 teaspoon baking soda

Directions:
- In a bowl, mix the almond flour with the coconut flesh, the zucchinis
- Add the other ingredients
- Stir well until you obtain a dough, shape 8 buns

Ingredients:
- ½ teaspoon cinnamon powder
- 3 tablespoons flaxseed mixed with
- 4 tablespoons water
- 1 cup coconut cream

- Arrange them on a baking sheet lined with parchment paper.
- Introduce in the oven at 350 degrees
- Bake for 30 minutes. Serve these sweet buns warm.

90) LIME CUSTARD

Preparation Time: 10 minutes **Cooking Time:** As per directions **Servings: 6**

Ingredients:
- 1 pint almond milk
- 4 tablespoons lime zest, grated
- 3 tablespoons lime juice

Directions:
- In a bowl, combine the almond milk with the lime zest, lime juice
- Add the other Ingredients

Ingredients:
- 3 tablespoons flaxseed mixed with
- 4 tablespoons water tablespoons stevia
- 2 teaspoons vanilla extract

- Whisk well and divide into 4 ramekins.
- Bake in the oven at 360 degrees F for 30 minutes.
- Cool the custard down and serve.

91) CANDIED PECANS

Preparation Time: 60 minutes   **Cooking Time:** As per directions   **Servings: 4**

Ingredients:
- 6 oz. Whole Pecans
- ½ cup Aquafaba
- 1 oz. Palm Sugar

Directions:
- Pre-heat oven to 350°F/180°C.
- Prepare a baking tray with a piece of parchment paper.
- Remove the cardamom seeds from the pods
- Crush the seeds and lay them onto one side of the tray.
- Chop the sugar or grind it in a food processor.
- Whisk the aquafaba until frothy

Ingredients:
- 1 oz. whole Green Cardamom Pods
- ¼ tsp. Salt
- 1 tsp. Allspice

- Stir in the sugar and salt
- Fold in the nuts, allspice, cardamom, until everything is coated.
- Spread the mixture evenly over the baking tray for about 15 minutes
- Replace it onto the cooling rack.
- When cooled, pecans can be enjoyed as a topping or as they are.

92) RICE AND CANTALOUPE RAMEKINS

Preparation Time: 10 minutes   **Cooking Time:** 30 minutes   **Servings: 4**

Ingredients:
- 2 tablespoons flaxseed mixed with
- 3 tablespoons water
- 2 cups cauliflower rice, steamed
- 1 cup coconut cream

Directions:
- In a bowl, mix the cauliflower rice with the flaxseed
- Mix and the other Ingredients except the cooking spray and whisk well.

Ingredients:
- 2 tablespoons stevia
- 1 teaspoon vanilla extract
- ½ cup cantaloupe, peeled and chopped
- Cooking spray

- Grease 4 ramekins with the cooking spray
- Divide the rice mix in each and cook at 360 degrees F for 30 minutes.
- Serve cold.

93) STRAWBERRIES CREAM

Preparation Time: 10 minutes   **Cooking Time:** 0 minutes   **Servings: 2**

Ingredients:
- 1 cup strawberries, chopped
- 1 cup coconut cream

Directions:
- In a blender, combine the strawberries with the cream

Ingredients:
- 1 tablespoon stevia
- ½ teaspoon vanilla extract

- Add the other ingredients
- Pulse well, divide into cups and serve cold.

94) ALMOND AND CHIA PUDDING

Preparation Time: 10 minutes   **Cooking Time:** 15 minutes   **Servings: 4**

Ingredients:
- 1 tablespoon lime juice
- 1 tablespoon lime zest, grated
- 2 cups almond milk
- 2 tablespoons almonds, chopped

Directions:
- In a pan, mix the almond milk with the chia seeds, the almonds
- Add the other ingredients

Ingredients:
- 1 teaspoon almond extract
- ½ cup chia seeds
- 2 tablespoons stevia

- Whisk, bring to a simmer
- Cook over medium heat for 15 minutes.
- Divide the mix into bowls and serve cold.

95) DATES AND COCOA BOWLS

Preparation Time: 2 hours   **Cooking Time:** 0 minutes   **Servings: 6**

Ingredients:
- 2 tablespoons avocado oil
- 1 cup coconut cream
- 1 teaspoon cocoa powder

Directions:
- In a bowl, mix the cream with the oil, the cocoa, the cream
- Add the other ingredients

Ingredients:
- ½ cup dates, chopped
- 3 tablespoons stevia

- Pulse well, divide into cups
- Keep in the fridge for 2 hours before serving.

96) NUTS AND SEEDS PUDDING

Preparation Time: 10 minutes   **Cooking Time:** 20 minutes   **Servings: 4**

Ingredients:
- 2 cups cauliflower rice
- ¼ cup coconut cream
- 2 cups almond milk
- 1 teaspoon vanilla extract

Directions:
- In a pan, combine the cauliflower rice with the cream, the almond milk
- Add the other ingredients

Ingredients:
- 3 tablespoons stevia
- ½ cup walnuts, chopped
- 1 tablespoon chia seeds
- Cooking spray

- Toss, bring to a simmer
- Cook over medium heat for 20 minutes.
- Divide into bowls and serve cold.

97) CASHEW FUDGE

Preparation Time: 3 hours **Cooking Time**: 0 minutes **Servings**: 6

Ingredients:
- 1/3 cup cashew butter
- 1 cup coconut cream
- ½ cup cashews, soaked for 8 hours and drained

Directions:
- In a bowl, mix the cashew butter with the cream, the cashews
- Add the other ingredients and whisk well.

Ingredients:
- 5 tablespoons lime juice
- ½ teaspoon lime zest, grated
- 1 tablespoons stevia
- Line a muffin tray with parchment paper, scoop 1 tablespoon of the fudge
- Mix in each of the muffin tins and freeze for 3 hours before serving.

98) LIME BERRIES STEW

Preparation Time: 10 minutes **Cooking Time**: 20 minutes **Servings**: 6

Ingredients:
- Zest of 1 lime, grated
- Juice of 1 lime
- 1 pint strawberries, halved

Directions:
- In a pan, combine the strawberries with the lime juice, the water and stevia

Ingredients:
- 2 cups water
- 2 tablespoons stevia
- Toss, bring to a simmer and cook over medium heat for 20 minutes.
- Divide the stew into bowls and serve cold.

99) APRICOTS CAKE

Preparation Time: 10 minutes **Cooking Time**: 30 minutes **Servings**: 8

Ingredients:
- ¾ cup stevia
- 2 cups coconut flour
- ¼ cup coconut oil, melted
- ½ cup almond milk
- 1 teaspoon baking powder

Directions:
- In a bowl, mix the flour with the coconut oil, the stevia
- Add the other ingredients
- Whisk and pour into a cake pan lined with parchment paper.

Ingredients:
- 2 tablespoons flaxseed mixed with 3 tablespoons water
- ½ teaspoon vanilla extract
- Juice of 1 lime
- 2 cups apricots, chopped
- Introduce in the oven at 375 degrees F
- Bake for 30 minutes, cool down, slice and serve.

100) BERRY CAKE

Preparation Time: 10 minutes **Cooking Time:** 30 minutes **Servings: 6**

Ingredients:
- 2 cups coconut flour
- 1 cup blueberries
- 1 cup strawberries, chopped
- 2 tablespoons almonds, chopped
- 2 tablespoons walnuts, chopped
- 3 tablespoons stevia
- 1 teaspoon almond extract

Ingredients:
- 3 tablespoons flaxseed mixed with
- 4 tablespoons water
- ½ cup coconut cream
- 2 tablespoons avocado oil
- 1 teaspoon baking powder
- Cooking spray

Directions:
- In a bowl, combine the coconut flour with the berries
- Add the nuts, stevia and the other ingredients, and whisk well.
- Grease a cake pan with the cooking spray, pour the cake mix inside
- Introduce everything in the oven at 360 degrees F
- Bake for 30 minutes. Cool the cake down, slice and serve.

Thanks for reading this book

CPSIA information can be obtained
at www.ICGtesting.com
Printed in the USA
BVHW051638140621
609528BV00009B/1312